IBS: *A* DOCTOR'S PLAN *for* CHRONIC DIGESTIVE TROUBLES

The Definitive Guide to Prevention and Relief

BY

GERARD GUILLORY, M.D.

HARTLEY & MARKS
PUBLISHERS

Published
in the U.S.A. by
Hartley & Marks, Inc.
Box 147, Point Roberts, WA
98281

Published
in Canada by
Hartley & Marks, Ltd.
3663 West Broadway
Vancouver, B.C.
V6R 2B8

Library of Congress Cataloging-In-Publication Data

Guillory, Gerard.
   IBS, a doctor's plan for chronic digestive troubles : the definitive guide to prevention and relief / by Gerard Guillory.
     p.   cm.
  Includes bibliographical references and index.
  ISBN 0-88179-031-1 : $11.95
  1. Irritable colon--Popular works.   I. Title.
RC862.I77G85   1991
616.3'44--dc20

91-13418
CIP

The ideas, methods, and suggestions in this book are not intended as a substitute for consultation with a physician

Cover design: Elizabeth Watson
The typeface is Janson, typeset by The Typeworks

TABLE OF CONTENTS

	Acknowledgements	vi
	Foreword	vii
	Introduction: The Truth about IBS	ix
Chapter 1	How IBS Affects You and How It Is Diagnosed	1
Chapter 2	Your Internal Food Processor	12
Chapter 3	Tracking Down Causes of IBS	17
Chapter 4	What You Should Know about the Role of Diet	21
Chapter 5	Tracking Down Problem Diet Factors	36
Chapter 6	Discovering the Value of High Fiber	50
Chapter 7	How Emotions Affect the Intestinal Tract	56
Chapter 8	The Importance of Proper Exercise	66
Chapter 9	Planning for Digestive Security	74
Chapter 10	Additional Tips for Treating Symptoms	89
Chapter 11	Important Facts about Medications	99
Chapter 12	For "Significant Others," about the Importance of Support	106
Chapter 13	Facts about Coexisting Conditions	114
Chapter 14	Other Common Gastrointestinal Disorders	122
Chapter 15	Common Tests You May Face	139
	Conclusion	150

Appendix 1   Questionnaires   151

Appendix 2   Common Questions and Answers about IBS   158

Appendix 3   All about Medication   164

Appendix 4   Lactose-Free Diet   181

Appendix 5   Foods High in Fiber   184

Appendix 6   How to Stop Smoking   186

Appendix 7   Making a Self-Relaxation Tape   189

             Glossary   192

             Further Reading   203

             Index   205

"Man should always strive to have his intestines relaxed all the days of his life." – MAIMONIDES, *12th-century physician*

The word "doctor" has its roots in the Latin word meaning "to teach," and patient education is an important aspect of the healing arts. As stated in the *American College of Physicians Ethos Manual*: "The patient should be informed and educated about his condition and should understand and approve of the treatment. In return, he should participate responsibly in his own care."

ACKNOWLEDGEMENTS

Although it is customary to acknowledge those who have contributed to an author's work, I do so with some trepidation as it is impossible to thank everyone who deserves my gratitude.

In many ways, the writing of this book has been an invaluable educational experience for me. I owe a great deal of thanks to my friend Mike Snipes, who helped me with many aspects of this project. From him I learned that the task was not overwhelming if it was divided into its component parts.

I would like to thank the many patients and physicians who responded to my request for input on a book about IBS. I owe a special thanks to Dr. Richard Fieman, Dr. Alan Fine, Dr. Joel Miller, and Dr. Richard Moore for their contributions. Mary Montgomery, Anthony Palmieri, and Dan Robinson from the Challenge Center contributed to the chapters on diet and exercise. Barbara Hansen and Nancy DeNiro from Aurora Presbyterian Hospital were most helpful with the section on tests used to evaluate the gastrointestinal tract. Sharon Martin, the hospital librarian, researched and provided every article I requested (no matter how obscure). Cynthia Brandes took over much of the typing and indexing for the book in the final critical stages.

My editor, Sue Tauber, and the staff at Hartley & Marks were a pleasure to work with. Sue, a psychologist, has keen insight into human nature and has herself become an expert in IBS.

A project like this would not be possible without the love, support, and encouragement of family members. My parents, both educators, provided a firm foundation for me and my siblings to pursue whatever dreams we had. My wife, Cheryll, spent many hours typing the initial pages as thoughts were put onto paper. I look forward to the extra time I shall have to spend with her now that this book is complete.

FOREWORD

It is my belief that Dr. Guillory has provided an important source of reference information for patients. The term "doctor" actually means teacher, derived from the Latin term "docere" — to teach. Teaching for and to medical students as they study to become physicians and continuing medical education for physicians in practice is a well-recognized teaching goal. Teaching patients to understand the principles of good health and to deal with health problems intelligently is, in my view, an equally important responsibility for the physician and is one which has not been as well met by the medical profession. And while other members of the health care team, nutritionists, pharmacists and nurse practitioners can help with patient education, the ultimate responsibility lies with the physician.

In the "good old days," physicians were apt to deal with patient concerns and questions in a paternalistic, sometimes patronizing fashion, leaving the patient with unanswered questions and anxieties, even though frequently the patient's problem was eventually "cured". No more! We live in an age of consumer activism. In medicine, patients want and frequently demand (rightly so) to know what the physician thinks might be wrong, what tests are being done and why, and what therapy is to be employed, and what options exist. Modern medicine has made remarkable strides in dealing with problems and diseases; much of the success has resulted from the application of complex technology both in the diagnosis and treatment of disease. Not only must physicians understand the application of these technologies, they must be able and willing to determine that the patient understands as well. Decisions concerning diagnosis and treatment require patient participation, and patients can intelligently participate only if they understand the issues involved. There are several ways in which patients can learn more and therefore make appropriate decisions. One of those ways is through the availability of written material done from the lay person's perspective and exemplified in Dr. Guillory's book. I would stress, however, that such material is intended only to complement patient understanding and should never be used as a guide to self-treatment or to replace appropriate medical care.

Of all the patient complaints seen by primary care physicians, those related to the gastrointestinal tract are the most common and amongst these, irritable bowel syndrome (IBS) is an especially important problem. As Dr. Guillory points out, the diagnosis of this problem is one of exclusion; there is no specific diagnostic test which confirms the diagnosis, so the physician relies on a careful history and the appropriate use of studies to exclude other, sometimes more serious disorders which can mimic IBS. The book is primarily intended for the intelligent lay reader and is written in an informal, though not patronizing style. You can literally feel the author's desire to help patients understand this perplexing problem. He begins with the definition of IBS and leads the reader through possible causes, or factors which may aggravate symptoms, emphasizing diet and emotions, and then discusses all aspects of the symptomatic treatment of the disease.

Of special value are the sections on other common gastrointestinal diseases which mimic IBS, and the diagnostic studies which may be required to exclude other diseases. The useful glossary explains much of the medical jargon in understandable terms. My hope is that patients who read this book will recieve hope and encouragement about management of the condition and that physicians will use it, and material like it, as they educate patients about the disease.

O'Neill Barrett, Jr, MD.
Chairman and Professor
Department of Medicine
University of South Carolina
School of Medicine

INTRODUCTION

THE TRUTH ABOUT IBS: IRRITABLE BOWEL SYNDROME,
SPASTIC COLON, SPASTIC COLITIS, MUCOUS COLITIS,
NERVOUS STOMACH, NERVOUS DIARRHEA,
FUNCTIONAL BOWEL DISEASE

The names may vary, but one fact is certain: suffering from this symptomatic disorder is no fun. It can cause embarrassment, create suspicion, harm relationships, shorten vacation trips, spoil parties, and turn gregarious people into recluses. The medical term most frequently used today is irritable bowel syndrome, or IBS, and there are still others that may represent variants of IBS, namely, esophageal spasm, aerophagia, nonulcer dyspepsia, and proctalgia fugax.

GENERAL SYMPTOMS AND PROBLEMS OF IBS

IBS is the most common of all digestive disorders, affecting as many as one in five adults in North America. This perplexing problem is the leading cause of chronic, recurrent abdominal pain, referred to as "gas pains" by some sufferers. The discomfort is linked with embarrassing symptoms such as sudden, unexpected bouts of diarrhea, belching, and excessive gas. Intermittent or chronic constipation is also common. People with uncontrolled IBS are rarely "regular"; their bowel movements tend to be either too fast or too slow.

I have listened with a sympathetic ear to countless stories of the annoyance, pain, and embarrassment caused by the symptoms. I have heard stories of shopping carts left unattended, of boardrooms awaiting the return of the presenter, of times of dire need when there was no change for the pay toilet. Then there was the desirable new date suddenly and mysteriously left alone several times during dinner, wondering what he may have done wrong. I recall the story of the college freshman who bolted from the classroom on several occasions during an exam "to relieve myself," leading the instructor to suspect that the student was hiding cheat sheets in the rest room.

Having IBS or spastic colon may mean going to an unfamiliar establishment and immediately having to locate the rest room in case you get an urgent call. It may mean acquainting yourself with all the rest stops along the route before you take an automobile trip. Female sufferers describe the anxiety of coping with long lines and jammed rest rooms at public events. "I won't go to a football game with my husband, because the fear of making it to the john is enough to trigger symptoms," one woman told me. The availability and accessibility of rest rooms becomes a major issue in life.

I am not certain the term "irritable bowel syndrome" is the most descriptive or even the most accurate. Perhaps "sensitive bowel syndrome" would be more in line with the symptoms and feelings of sufferers. "Irritable bowel syndrome" has negative connotations that make sufferers feel that they, somehow, are personally responsible for their condition. As you will see in later chapters, the specific cause remains unknown and there is, as yet, no final cure.

The fact is, the majority of the population can eat and drink as it pleases, without suffering intense cramps and altered patterns of bowel movements. Those with IBS have guts that are "sensitive" to various edibles (triggers) that the average person tolerates without difficulty. However, marked improvement *is* possible.

PROFILE OF AN IBS SUFFERER

In my experience treating those suffering from IBS, I can say that there is no exclusive profile of a person with this disorder. Single, married, student, professional, craftsperson, home-maker—all can be affected. Some are unaware that they suffer from IBS; others have come to believe their abnormal bowel function is without remedy, and thus no longer seek qualified medical treatment.

For example, I first saw Adrean after she had had a moped accident while she was on vacation. While I was obtaining a background medical history, she said that she had experienced problems with her colon most of her adult life. And since the accident, she had experienced worsening abdominal pain and diarrhea. At this point, it became apparent that her digestive problems were more troublesome to her than the bumps and bruises she had sustained.

After concluding that her problems did indeed stem from IBS, we began a combined approach emphasizing diet, stress reduction, and medications. After several months, Adrean's condition had improved, and she became instrumental in forming an educational/support group for IBS patients.

DIAGNOSING AND TREATING IBS

Fortunately, there is hope. I have found that many people respond favorably to a combination of treatments and are thus able to rediscover normal daily and social activities that may previously have been difficult or impossible as a result of IBS.

This book is not intended to replace the diagnosis or treatment of IBS, which should only be performed by a physician. The intent of this book is to offer you insights and guidelines for dealing with the complexities of this problem. I advise you to use it as an aid to living with IBS and to enlist the help and guidance of a sympathetic medical practitioner. When you see your physician, I recommend bringing along a completed copy of the diet diary and the questionnaire from Appendix 1. And IBS sufferers will find it much easier to gain support when they share Chapter 12, "For 'Significant Others,' about the Importance of Support," with concerned loved ones.

Although the exact cause of IBS remains unknown, several theories regarding possible causes have been developed. Poor dietary habits in general, specific food sensitivities, lack of dietary fiber, and emotional stress are among the many factors implicated. Whatever the cause, research has shown that IBS symptoms occur with irregular movement of gastrointestinal contents through the digestive system, and certain interruptions in the rhythm of movement are suspected of setting off the symptoms. The greatest success in treating symptoms comes from following an established approach to diagnosis and treatment of any disease: establishing the diagnosis; searching for aggravating factors; recommending appropriate lifestyle changes; judiciously using medications, if needed; and projecting an expected outcome.

The first step, establishing the diagnosis, is probably the most important one. For some people, a diagnosis can be difficult to make, as symptoms may differ from those of the classic case. They may present a confusing picture to the physician, who then may believe that extensive testing is warranted. Others may come with textbook symptoms and obvious triggers that when avoided lead to prompt resolution of symptoms. When this happens, exhaustive testing may not be necessary. Thus, the length of time it will take to establish a diagnosis of IBS and to find effective treatment will often vary a great deal.

Unfortunately, many people have come to me only after attempting to treat themselves with over-the-counter remedies for their diarrhea, constipation, or abdominal pain, before being systematically evaluated for the cause of these symptoms. Before treating these symptoms, it is most important to discover their cause. Establishing the diagnosis is described in detail in Chapter 1, "How ibs Affects You and How It Is Diagnosed."

The second step is to check for aggravating factors. For instance, I have found that many people with ibs symptoms have a coexisting dairy product (lactose) intolerance. Avoiding dairy products or using lactase enzyme supplements has often led to resolution or a marked improvement of symptoms in this group. In addition, hidden food sensitivities, improper exercise, other poor lifestyle habits, and stress can each aggravate digestive problems.

The third step is to make significant changes in your lifestyle. This step is calculated to help individuals become as healthy as they can possibly be and involves five basic areas: proper diet; exercise; stress reduction; moderation in daily living; finding a social sense of well-being.

The World Health Organization (who) has defined health as the complete stage of mental, physical, and social well-being. Although I have not encountered anyone who has been able to totally achieve this stage, it is certainly a worthwhile goal.

Lack of exercise, stress, and poor dietary habits can have direct effects on the digestive tract. These factors may also lead to such problems as hypertension, diabetes, and obesity. In turn, such disorders and the medications taken to treat them may adversely affect the gut. Thus, by taking steps to ensure your general health, you will be better able to ensure your digestive health as well.

To have a social sense of well-being means to feel comfortable in social situations. Finding a social sense of well-being is important, because it helps to enhance the self-esteem necessary to prevent depression and anxiety. You should feel good about who you are and why you are here; this attitude will give you a positive sense of control over your life and prevent mood disorders, which may lead to overeating or lack of appetite.

IBS is symptomatic. That is, we recognize the disorder in a set of symptoms. Not all sufferers experience identical symptoms, a factor that clouds instant diagnosis. The theory is, treat the symptoms, and the disorder will often lapse into remission.

And practice generally confirms this theory.

Theresa was perhaps the last person anyone would expect to see in a doctor's office. She was young and, on the surface, appeared very healthy. A member of a local health club, she worked out regularly, was in good physical condition, and was very diet conscious. On her first visit to me, she complained of a "burning pain" in the pit of her stomach, and bowel movements that were either too loose or too hard. " I never seem to have a regular bowel movement," she said.

These symptoms first appeared, I discovered, shortly after a promotion at work and usually occurred during times of stress, particularly while Theresa was at work. I first obtained an X ray of the upper gastrointestinal tract to rule out an ulcer and made a tentative diagnosis of IBS. We also discussed Theresa's lack of self-confidence, particularly in her new position at work. After she had explored this idea, she was able to help herself through simple assertiveness training.

Today Theresa has her symptoms well under control as a result of her changed attitude about herself. She is on her way to achieving an enhanced state of mental, physical, and social well-being. For Theresa, treating the symptoms had a great deal to do with the way she perceived herself and her worth.

You may not necessarily need attention in all five areas, but if you want to be as healthy as possible, analyze your personal situation to determine the areas in which you may need to improve. Some changes may be as simple as 20 minutes of exercise three times a week and watching your intake of certain food groups. Other changes may be more complicated, and take more time, and what works for you may not work for someone else.

The fourth step in treating IBS symptoms, the judicious use of medications, is employed only after aggravating factors have been eliminated and appropriate lifestyle changes made without the complete removal of symptoms.

The final step in this approach to diagnosis and treatment is to project an expected outcome. Whereas a percentage of IBS sufferers experience spontaneous remission and become virtually symptom free, for the majority, recurring symptoms will remain a concern. The primary goal is to help you live successfully with this disorder, minimizing symptoms as much as possible. It is important for you to realize this so that you will not become discouraged if your symptoms recur after a long symptom-free interval.

THE IMPORTANCE OF EDUCATION

The more people know about a particular disorder, the better they are able to cope with the problem. I therefore place great emphasis on education as an aspect of treatment and view patient education as one of the most important and challenging aspects of medical practice. The physician must become teacher as well as diagnostician and clinician.

My first personal appreciation of patient education came when I was a fourth-year medical student doing a clinical clerkship in a small, indigent hospital. The hospital employed a social worker whose full-time job was to educate patients about their medical conditions. The result was better-informed patients who were more likely to comply with medical advice and more likely to improve.

During my training, I helped write patient educational literature and have continued to write such materials after beginning my own medical practice. I now see how a well-informed person stands a much better chance of doing well and cooperating in his or her own healing than one who is uninformed and simply enduring treatment.

BREAKING THE TABOO

IBS is not new, but I truly believe it is becoming more prevalent. Our hurry-up lifestyles emphasizing early achievement and super-success clearly foster unbearable stresses, poor eating habits, and little time to nurture one's self-esteem. For those who are predisposed to develop IBS, modern lifestyles create the "perfect" environment to cultivate this disorder.

At this point, you may be wondering why, if IBS is so common, you haven't heard more about it. The fact is that the topic of our bowel functions arises only infrequently during everyday conversation. It is as if this subject is too personal, making its discussion taboo. When the topic *is* discussed, it is most often the source of a good laugh. An IBS sufferer, however, is not likely to find the subject humorous.

Fortunately, IBS has recently been receiving long-overdue attention in medical literature. I resolved to write a small guide for IBS sufferers when I could find no comprehensive text that adequately covered the topic. That first attempt received enthusiastic response and evoked valuable comment from both physicians and patients. I was encouraged by the number of patients who found relief by following the advice in my book. Many, however, also posed good questions that had not been adequately addressed. The information I received at that time made me decide to broaden the scope of the initial work. In addition, much new information and many new treatments are emerging, and I have incorporated them into this book.

I hope you find the information and recommendations contained in this edition helpful, and I invite your comments or suggestions to help improve future editions. (Please refer to the note at the end of the book.)

1

HOW IBS AFFECTS YOU

AND

HOW IT IS DIAGNOSED

Irritable bowel syndrome, or IBS, has had several names in the past, the most common of which is spastic colon. Other terms have included "spastic colitis," "mucous colitis," and "nervous stomach." Since "colitis" implies inflammation of the colon—and since IBS involves no inflammation and is not limited to the colon—this term is generally no longer used. "Irritable bowel syndrome," in contrast, implies an irritability of the entire bowel. A syndrome is a group of symptoms or signs that occur together and produce a pattern typical of a particular disorder. Thus, irritable bowel syndrome is a group of symptoms involving the entire digestive tract, the alimentary canal.

Irritable bowel syndrome was first described in North America in 1817, and several papers on it appeared in English literature beginning the following year. These early accounts emphasized passage of "membranes" in the stool, perhaps because only the most severe examples were recognized, and because most cases reported involved the abuse of purgatives or enemas.

Physicians often refer to IBS as a functional disorder, with abnormal functioning of the gastrointestinal tract but without identifiable structural damage. General agreement is that it results from disordered movement of the gastrointestinal tract. Normal rhythmic contractions are somehow interrupted, much as the heart may beat abnormally.

SYMPTOMS OF IBS

Classic IBS symptoms include abdominal pain, together with an altered pattern of defecation. Abdominal pain is the most frequent complaint of IBS sufferers, and the pain patterns are quite diverse. Different sufferers describe it as aching, crampy, burning, or sharp. The pains can be relatively constant but are more commonly intermittent. The defecation pattern may consist of constipation, or diarrhea, or a pattern of constipation alternating with diarrhea.

The urge to have a bowel movement is often sudden and is experienced along with a crampy pain that is relieved after the passage of feces or gas. After the bowel movement, there may be a sense of incomplete evacuation, as if there were a fullness in the rectum, suggesting evacuation is not finished.

Often people complain of belching, bloating, nausea, decreased appetite, and excessive gas. Researchers have described other characteristics that may not involve the gut but that are found to occur more frequently in IBS sufferers than in the normal population. These include frequency of urination, incomplete emptying of the bladder, an unpleasant taste in the mouth, fatigue, and uncomfortable intercourse in women. For some undetermined reason, IBS occurs twice as frequently in women as men in North America. In India and Sri Lanka, however, estimates show a higher incidence of IBS in males than females. One possible explanation is that there are cultural factors that determine who seeks medical care, and these cultural factors are more important than sex.

There are estimates that fewer than half of those suffering from IBS in North America report their complaint to a physician. Some people may have multiple medical complaints, including bowel complaints, and they may be more inclined to discuss those aches, pains, and concerns that they find less embarrassing. For example, IBS seems to occur more commonly in stress-prone individuals, and they often exhibit other manifestations of stress, including tension headaches, dizziness, fatigue, diffuse muscular aches, palpitations, chest pain, and tingling of the hands and feet.

IBS symptoms commonly coexist with various other disorders. For example, you may experience them in conjunction with premenstrual syndrome (PMS) or with fibromyalgia syndrome (FMS). FMS is a disorder of unknown cause, characterized by generalized aching and stiffness. The major symptoms of these two disorders may predominate and prompt you to consult your physician. You should take care to discuss the disordered bowel function in addition to the other symptoms, which may overshadow the intestinal complaint. (See Chapter 13, "Facts about Coexisting Conditions," for a complete discussion of premenstrual syndrome and fibromyalgia syndrome.)

DIAGNOSING IBS

The approach to diagnosing IBS varies with a person's age, duration of his or her symptoms, and the most prevalent symptoms experienced. In addition, physicians may vary somewhat in their approach to problem solving. Unfortunately, there is no single conclusive test available to diagnose IBS.

I begin the diagnosis with what I consider the most important first step: a detailed clinical history followed by a physical exam. Then I order a limited number of routine screening tests. I may order blood tests, a urinalysis, and a stool specimen test to check for blood in the stool or for bowel infection. There may be other, more specialized tests, to exclude the presence of any diseases or pathological disorders suggested by the history and exam. These procedures are followed in order to exclude other diseases or disorders that may produce similar symptoms. For example, I ordered an upper gastrointestinal (upper GI) X ray for

Theresa to rule out an ulcer as the cause of the burning pain she reported.

For others, more thorough testing may be necessary. Charles, a 55-year-old college professor, complained of worsening constipation and sharp abdominal pains. His medical history revealed a lot of "colic" while he was growing up, although he had been free of symptoms for many years. Because of his age and his symptoms, I suggested both a colon X ray and a sigmoid exam (direct observation of the colon with a fiberoptic instrument), to exclude the possibility of colon cancer. When these tests returned normal, I recommended a gradual increase in dietary fiber. Charles has since done quite well.

Others, by the nature of the discomforts, may warrant gallbladder tests or direct visual inspection of the digestive tract by endoscopy. When all tests prove inconclusive, or when I see a patient who I believe is suffering from IBS but who is not responding to treatment, I may refer him or her to a gastroenterologist for a second opinion. As an internist, I often consult with other specialists in their respective disciplines.

Gastroenterologists are physicians who specialize in the treatment of digestive disorders. I will refer a patient for a second opinion if I am unsure of the diagnosis, or if there is or has been unsatisfactory response to treatment. Conversely, if I am confident of the diagnosis and the patient is feeling well, referral is not necessary. In addition, gastroenterologists are trained to do the specialized tests that may be required when a diagnosis of IBS is not clear.

CHOOSING A DOCTOR

You may or may not be under the care of a physician for your bowel complaints. If not, I encourage you to find one. Whom should you see? How do you choose a doctor? These are important questions that need to be addressed.

The best time to choose a doctor is before you urgently need one. Choosing a doctor before an emergency occurs allows you the opportunity to do some research into the doctor's qualifications and references, the nature of the practice, office hours, hospital affiliations, and so on. Ask those you trust to suggest a physician, or ask if they know anything about a doctor you are considering. Many local hospitals and medical societies have physician-referral services. See if you can set up a brief "get-acquainted" visit with the doctor you have chosen. (The initial charge, if any, will be well spent in the long run.)

Another question is whether you should see a specialist. I suggest you first see a primary-care physician (family practitioner, internist, or pediatrician). Odds are that he or she will be able to suggest an effective evaluation and treatment plan. If you are not given a treatment plan to address your symptoms, ask your primary-care physician to recommend a gastroenterologist. Many specialists prefer—or may even require—that you have an established primary-care physician. The primary-care physician is in a better position to treat the whole patient, focusing not only on the digestive system but on the interrelationship of all body systems as well. If you are a woman, you may have an established relationship with an obstetrician/gynecologist, with whom you can discuss your digestive disorder to obtain recommendations regarding evaluation, treatment, or referral.

There are some important things you can do before the first visit to help your doctor gather useful information about your digestive problem. The most important step in establishing a diagnosis of IBS is to obtain a detailed clinical history. Many medical authorities now contend that a correct diagnosis can often be made based entirely on the sufferer's historical account of symptoms. This is fortunate, since it may make extensive testing unnecessary. This is not to say that certain tests may not be required to rule out other disorders. Common tests used to evaluate the gastrointestinal tract are discussed in Chapter 15, "Common Tests You May Face," and Chapter 14, "Other Common Gastrointestinal Disorders," describes other common gastrointestinal conditions.

5

At the end of this chapter are some questions that have been found of great value to my patients. Take an active role by writing down the answers to these questions before you visit the doctor. Part I consists of questions about your digestive problem, and Part II consists of questions about your general medical history and background. Although the list is relatively long, each question is important, because it will tend to either suggest or exclude one of the many potential causes of your symptoms. This list may be photocopied and filled in to take with you on your first visit to the doctor. Although the list is not exhaustive, and your physician may ask you to answer additional questions, it will serve as a useful framework to help characterize your symptoms. A detailed account of other medical problems, medications, dietary history, family history, and seemingly unrelated symptoms is also important for your physician to gain a complete understanding of all factors in planning for your diagnosis and treatment.

SUMMARY

Since IBS was first described, it has also been called spastic colon, spastic colitis, mucous colitis, and nervous stomach, among other names.

Symptoms include abdominal pain associated with an altered pattern of defecation. Some sufferers complain of belching, bloating, nausea, decreased appetite, and excessive gas.

Whereas IBS is only an occasional nuisance for some, others find that the symptoms interfere with many aspects of their daily lives.

IBS often coexists with other disorders.

The diagnosis will vary with a person's age, the duration of symptoms, and prevalent symptoms.

Determining IBS includes a detailed clinical history and a physical exam, which may be followed by screening tests to exclude diseases or disorders suggested by the examination and history.

DIAGNOSTIC QUESTIONS

PART I

1. How long have you had abdominal pain?
2. Do you have more than one pain? Yes ☐   No ☐
   If so, how many different pains do you have?
3. Where is the worst pain located?
4. How often does the pain occur, and how long does it generally last?
5. Does the pain ever awaken you from sleep?
6. Is the pain ever so severe that it is unbearable and interferes with your normal daily activities?
7. How would you describe the pain? Cramping, aching, burning, knifelike, or... ?
8. Have you found anything you can do or take to alleviate the pain?
9. Does eating or drinking make the pain better or worse?
10. Have you identified certain foods that seem to trigger pain or diarrhea?
11. Describe your typical pattern of bowel movements and the consistency of feces. (For example, one bowel movement, every three days, which is hard and difficult to pass, or two or three loose, watery bowel movements a day.)
12. Has this pattern remained constant, or has it changed in recent months?
13. Is the pain usually relieved after a bowel movement?
14. Are the bowel movements more loose or more frequent after the onset of pain?
15. Do you have any of the following associated symptoms? (Circle those that apply to you.)
    a. Bloating
    b. Belching
    c. Gas
    d. Nausea
    e. Vomiting

16. Have you lost weight in recent months? If so, how much over what time period?
17. Have you passed blood in your stool or had black, tarry bowel movements?
18. Have you previously been evaluated for these complaints? If so, what tests were performed, and what were the results?
19. Comment on the effectiveness or side effects of any previously prescribed medications that you have taken for your complaints.

PART II

SMOKER: Yes ☐   No ☐
Packs per day _____
For how many years? _____
If a former smoker, when did you quit? _____

ALCOHOL: Yes ☐   No ☐
Drinks per week (average) _____
Have you ever felt guilty about the amount you drink or have you ever felt a need to control your drinking? Yes ☐   No ☐

CAFFEINE: Cups of coffee per day _____
Other (tea, cola, etc.) _____

MEDICATIONS: List medications, prescription and nonprescription, taken regularly. Please include dosage, frequency, and how long you have taken them.

_____
_____
_____

ALLERGIES: List allergies and type of reaction (e.g., penicillin—rash)

_____
_____

Please list those medical problems that your immediate family members have or had. If deceased, list the age and cause of death if known (e.g., father—high blood pressure, deceased age 50—heart attack)

_____

_____

_____

RATE YOUR OVERALL HEALTH
Poor ☐   Fair ☐   Good ☐   Excellent ☐

EXERCISE: Do you exercise regularly? Yes ☐   No ☐
If yes, describe the types of exercise and frequency:

_____

_____

_____

NUTRITION AND DIET:
How many meals do you eat each day? _____
Do you usually eat breakfast? Yes ☐   No ☐
Do you diet frequently and/or are you now dieting? Yes ☐ No ☐
Do you eat, for you, a balanced diet?
Almost always ☐   Sometimes ☐   Rarely ☐

LIST ANY FOOD SUPPLEMENTS OR VITAMINS YOU TAKE REGULARLY:

_____

_____

_____

DO YOU HAVE OR HAVE YOU EVER BEEN TREATED FOR ANY OF THE FOLLOWING? Please check yes or no. If you check yes, please give date of treatment or occurrence.

	YES	DATE	NO
Asthma or wheezing	☐	_____	☐
Hayfever or allergies	☐	_____	☐

9

	Yes	Date	No
Tuberculosis	☐	_____	☐
Chronic or persistent cough	☐	_____	☐
Chronic chest condition	☐	_____	☐
Frequent colds, sinus or nose trouble	☐	_____	☐
Stomach or duodenal ulcers	☐	_____	☐
Persistent or recurrent indigestion	☐	_____	☐
Bowel or intestinal trouble	☐	_____	☐
Gallbladder stones or colic	☐	_____	☐
Liver trouble or jaundice	☐	_____	☐
Dysentery or colitis	☐	_____	☐
Rectal trouble or bleeding	☐	_____	☐
Diabetes or sugar in urine	☐	_____	☐
Kidney trouble	☐	_____	☐
High blood pressure or hypertension	☐	_____	☐
Heart trouble, murmurs, or heart attack	☐	_____	☐
Chest pain	☐	_____	☐
Shortness of breath	☐	_____	☐
Chronic or recurrent eye trouble	☐	_____	☐
Chronic or recurrent ear trouble	☐	_____	☐
Any birth abnormalities	☐	_____	☐
Fatigue	☐	_____	☐
Insomnia	☐	_____	☐
Snoring	☐	_____	☐
Serious bodily injury	☐	_____	☐
Rheumatism or arthritis	☐	_____	☐
Rheumatic fever	☐	_____	☐
Swollen or painful joints	☐	_____	☐
Backache or back injury	☐	_____	☐
Rupture or hernia	☐	_____	☐
Skin disease, rash, or acne	☐	_____	☐
Fainting spells	☐	_____	☐
Stroke	☐	_____	☐
Paralysis	☐	_____	☐
Epilepsy, seizures, convulsions	☐	_____	☐

	YES	DATE	NO
Varicose veins	☐	_____	☐
Piles or hemorrhoids	☐	_____	☐
Painful or difficult urination	☐	_____	☐
Hypoglycemia	☐	_____	☐
Goiter or thyroid trouble	☐	_____	☐
High metabolism	☐	_____	☐
Low metabolism	☐	_____	☐
Cancer	☐	_____	☐
Anemia	☐	_____	☐
Protein, blood, or pus in urine	☐	_____	☐
Frequent headaches	☐	_____	☐
Migraine headaches	☐	_____	☐
Alcohol addiction	☐	_____	☐
Drug addiction	☐	_____	☐
Sexual problems	☐	_____	☐

HOSPITAL ADMISSIONS FOR: SURGERY, INJURY, OR MATERNITY

Diagnosis   Mo/Year   Hospital/City   Physician

_____

_____

_____

FEMALE PATIENTS ONLY

Menstrual cycles began at age _____
Date of last period _____
Describe any menstrual irregularity:

_____

_____

Total number of pregnancies _____
Total number of miscarriages or abortions _____
Have you gone through menopause? Yes ☐   No ☐
If yes, at what age? _____
Do you take calcium supplements? Yes ☐   No ☐

11

2

YOUR INTERNAL
FOOD PROCESSOR

Digestion works like a giant food processor, using both mechanical and chemical means to break down the food you eat into elements suitable for your body to use. Our digestive system consists of the alimentary canal and its glands. In its most basic sense, the alimentary canal is a hollow tube some 27 feet long. In the 15 to 72 hours it takes a meal to pass through, the alimentary canal adds chemicals and hormones, mixes well, extracts nutrients and water, and reserves the refuse for elimination.

THE ROLE OF THE BRAIN

Your brain is the first organ involved in digestion, and just the thought, sight, or smell of food is enough for it to initiate the secretion of digestive juices and saliva. I recall coming home from college during the holidays, walking through the front door, and beginning to salivate in anticipation of the usual Thanksgiving feast. I am certain the digestive juices began flowing as soon as I encountered the first whiff of roasting turkey that permeated our house. By the time I sat down at the table, my "food processor" was primed and ready to go.

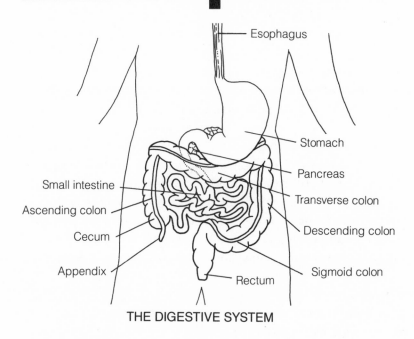

THE DIGESTIVE SYSTEM

CHEWING

As soon as you take a bite of food, you begin the second phase of digestion: chewing. Chewing has several functions: it tears the food into smaller pieces for easier swallowing, exposes a greater surface to digestive fluids, and mixes it with saliva and mucin. Chewing and swallowing, incidentally, are the only conscious acts of digestion. After that, the autonomic nervous system takes over and you're on automatic pilot.

Most of us chew too little and swallow too fast. Oriental medicine suggests that you chew each mouthful up to 50 times to complete this important phase of digestion.

Dentists have observed that the oral cavity must be in optimal operating order to ensure proper function. Peridontal disease, developmental abnormalities, poorly fitting dentures, or mechanical injury of your teeth, jaw, and supporting structures can lead to inadequate or painful chewing. If your ability to chew food is impaired, consider a dental evaluation and take any necessary steps to correct problems.

SWALLOWING

When you swallow, your esophagus—the portion of the alimentary canal between your mouth and stomach—propels each bolus, or portion of food, to your waiting stomach. The act of swallowing involves an action known as peristalsis, in which the muscles of your esophagus establish a wavelike rhythm of contractions that propel the bolus along its way, much like squeezing a toothpaste tube causes toothpaste to move through the tube and eventually squirt out. This action is so efficient that you can swallow even when you are upside down. Some of the problems encountered with IBS or "nervous stomach" stem from an interruption in the normal timing and rhythmical action of peristalsis.

MOVING FOOD THROUGH THE STOMACH AND INTESTINES

The stomach, which is the widest portion of the alimentary canal, serves as a sort of waiting room and preparation chamber. The stomach releases acids to assist in breaking down food particles; it also releases mucus to protect the stomach lining from acid burns. The stomach continues a rhythmical movement to mix the food with stomach acid, turning the food into a semi-digested material called chyme.

Through peristaltic movement, successive amounts of chyme enter the first part of the small intestine, called the duodenum. The small intestine is so named because of its diameter. It is actually some 21 feet long and extends from the stomach to the large intestine.

In the duodenum, chyme comes into contact with enzymes from the pancreas and bile from the gallbladder. The pancreas produces the enzymes protease, amylase and lipase. These assist, respectively, in breaking down proteins into amino acids, complex carbohydrates into simple sugars, and fat into fatty acids.

Bile is manufactured in the liver and stored in the gallbladder. It acts as an emulsifier by dividing fats into smaller particles that will become suspended in water. This allows fats—which do not mix well with water—to be more easily absorbed, in the same way that detergents break up grease. Bile acids are a constituent of bile and may be irritating to the intestines. In some people, excessive bile acids may enter the intestinal tract, causing diarrhea. This is fairly common in patients who have recently had a cholecystectomy (surgical removal of the gallbladder). There are specific medications that bind bile acids and can help such patients. (See Appendix 3 for more information.)

The small intestine contains many folds and fingerlike projections called "villi." Villi absorb the component parts of chyme—amino acids, simple sugars, and fatty acids—and pass them through the bloodstream into the liver for additional modification and use throughout your body. Indigestible parts of your food move from the small intestine into the large intestine.

The large intestine, or colon, is approximately three feet long and consists of the cecum, ascending colon, transverse colon, descending colon, sigmoid, and rectum. Although these names refer to different segments of the large intestine, it functions as a unit, absorbing excess water and storing digestive by-products until elimination.

The normal rhythm of peristalsis moves food along the entire digestive system. When this normal action is interrupted by such factors as diet or emotional stress, the result is often the discomfort experienced by those suffering from spastic colon or IBS.

SUMMARY

Digestion breaks down the food you eat into elements suitable for bodily use. Such factors as poor diet and emotional stress interrupt this process and contribute to the discomfort known as IBS.

The brain is the first organ to be involved in digestion, preparing the body to receive nourishment.

Chewing and swallowing are the only conscious acts of digestion. The esophagus propels food through the stomach with a rhythmic movement known as peristalsis. In the stomach, acids assist in breaking down food particles into a substance called chyme. Chyme moves through the small and large intestines, where digestive by-products are stored for elimination.

3

TRACKING DOWN
CAUSES OF IBS

I once attended a medical lecture on high blood pressure. After the lecture, a physician in the audience posed a very thought-provoking question to the guest speaker, a visitor from a prestigious medical university.

The speaker paused briefly, then replied, "That is a very good question. If I were a medical student, I would answer, 'I don't know.' As a professor of medicine, I must state, 'The answer is not known.' "

It is the same for the question "What causes irritable bowel syndrome?" The answer is not known. We understand what happens; we just don't have a complete understanding of *why* it happens.

Several causes of IBS have been suggested. Three of these are lack of dietary fiber, abnormal responses of the gastrointestinal tract to emotional stress, and specific food intolerance or sensitivities. As it turns out, all three may be causes to varying degrees in different people.

In fact, some authorities have divided patients into subgroups called "food reactors," "psychological reactors," and "mixed reactors." One authority states that "irritable bowel syndrome is not likely to be a single disorder, but rather a spectrum of disorders resulting from disturbances at all levels of the gut."

DISORDERED RHYTHM IN THE GASTROINTESTINAL TRACT

So although the exact cause of IBS is unknown, and it is unlikely that there is a single cause for the disorder, the common denominator among sufferers seems to be a disordered rhythm in the gastrointestinal tract. Let me explain. As described in Chapter 2, "Your Internal Food Processor," normal movement of intestinal contents depends on the orderly contractile rhythm of the intestinal smooth muscle—the movement known as peristalsis. Problems arise with disruption of this natural rhythm of bowel muscle, and these are known as IBS.

Intestinal contractions consist of "segmental contractions" (which essentially mix and churn intestinal contents), and "propulsive contractions" (which move intestinal contents forward). During periods of exaggerated segmental contractions, someone may experience abdominal cramps, bloating, and constipation. Forward movement decreases, and the stools become hard and compressed, making them difficult to pass.

Imagine, for a moment, that you are holding in both hands a long, thin balloon and that this balloon represents a portion of your intestinal tract. Suddenly, you squeeze with both hands— and the center of the balloon bulges. This is similar to what happens when segmented contractions are amplified, and this produces painful cramps or spasms.

Exaggerated propulsive contractions lead to bowel movements that are loose and frequent. People with this condition may also feel a sense of urgency, experiencing a sudden need for a bowel movement, as they frantically search for the nearest rest room.

In some ways, IBS or a spastic colon is analogous to asthma. In fact, IBS has been referred to as "asthma of the bowel." Like the hollow intestinal tract, the hollow bronchial breathing tubes contain sheets of smooth muscle fibers. Various stimuli, including emotional stress, inhaled irritants, and food substances, can trigger contractions of bronchial smooth muscle, resulting in breathlessness and wheezing.

FACTORS THAT TRIGGER SYMPTOMS

Everyone's digestive system functions a little differently, and there are various factors that may trigger symptoms in any given individual. These factors include the timing and content of meals, stressful situations, and various hormones. For example, eating a meal that is high in fat (like fried chicken) stimulates the release of a hormone called cholecystokinin. Cholecystokinin is, among other things, a potent stimulus for propulsive contractions of the colon. In some cases, I believe that this may account for worsening symptoms immediately after ingestion of a fatty meal.

Stress may also lead to exacerbated IBS symptoms by disturbing the intestine's motility. Common examples are the "butterflies in the stomach" or "nervous diarrhea" that most people have, at some time, experienced before moments of high stress. For a detailed discussion of how emotions can affect the intestinal tract, see Chapter 7, "How Emotions Affect the Intestinal Tract."

Some researchers have suggested that symptoms of IBS develop as the result of "learned illness behavior"; adults who now have IBS were given special consideration and "treats" when they experienced abdominal pain as children. Almost half of those with recurrent abdominal pain in childhood had symptoms of IBS 30 years later. These studies suggest that there may be psychological factors, with origins during childhood, that perpetuate symptoms of IBS. My own observations suggest that it is difficult to determine whether and how much psychological and physical factors contribute to the development of symptoms.

The key is to realize that psychological factors or emotional stress, and physical factors, such as food sensitivities, often must both be investigated in tracking down causes of IBS.

The following chapters cover the effects of proper diet, fiber, and food sensitivities, and how to effectively deal with emotional stress. If you have a spastic colon, you are the specialist for your particular symptoms. However, you should see your physician, because he or she is the specialist who can determine which mechanisms may underlie your symptoms. Only by working together will you be able to discover what is causing irritable bowel syndrome in your particular case.

SUMMARY

No exact cause of IBS, or spastic colon, is known; it is unlikely there is a single cause.

People are often classified as food reactors, psychological reactors, and mixed reactors.

Problems arise when the natural rhythms of the contractions in the intestines are disrupted.

Every digestive system is different and reacts differently to such things as timing and content of meals, stressful situations, and the releasing of various hormones. Stress may also exacerbate existing IBS symptoms.

4

WHAT YOU SHOULD KNOW

ABOUT

THE ROLE OF DIET

We all need proper nutrition for our general good health, but proper nutrition is absolutely essential for those with chronic digestive disorders, such as IBS, or spastic colon. Your body responds automatically when you eat. In fact, it must react to the meal so as to set in motion the normal digestive process, which allows your body to extract the nutrients it needs. Eating, for most, is one of life's greater pleasures. However, for those suffering from IBS, it can be a painful, annoying experience. This chapter presents general dietary recommendations that I hope will help you understand how certain foods may cause pain and other unpleasant symptoms.

RECIPE FOR INDIGESTION

Warren is an important publishing executive. His days are filled with deadlines, and there are never enough hours in a day to meet them all. He rushes out to lunch, taking a sheaf of contracts with him, and orders hastily from a menu in a crowded café. He drinks coffee while he waits. "If I could only dispense with the time it takes to eat," he thinks, "I would have time to review the Thompson proposal before that meeting in ten minutes." When his sandwich arrives, he devours it, while concentrating on the presentation, and washes it down with iced tea, followed by more coffee and a cigarette. Then, to freshen his breath, he pops a stick of gum into his mouth.

An hour and a half later, Warren returns from the meeting to his office. There are telephone messages to be answered and more paperwork to take care of as a result of the meeting. He has indigestion and a bloated, crampy, abdominal pain. And no wonder!

It is important to understand that although some foods may be bothersome, it is often the way they are eaten, rather than the specific food, that aggravates symptoms.

RULES TO EAT BY

Attempt to set aside enough time to eat so that you have the opportunity to dine in an unhurried, relaxed atmosphere. Take time to properly chew your food. Chewing makes the whole remainder of the digestive process easier, allowing your digestive tract to function as it was designed to function. As you may recall, chewing is the only aspect of the digestive process over which you routinely exercise conscious control. (Digestion is unconsciously controlled by the automatic nervous system, which responds to deep-breathing techniques and autohypnosis. See Chapter 7, "How Emotions Affect the Intestinal Tract.")

Chances are you would not attempt to place a raw carrot in your stomach without chewing, but even if you are eating well-cooked, puréed carrots, you should still take the time to eat slowly. This allows the digestive enzymes from the salivary glands to mix with the food. Those eating too quickly also often swallow an excessive amount of air (aerophagia), ending up with a bloated feeling. So the first advice to Warren would be to take advantage of this conscious aspect of digestion: eat slowly and chew your food well.

Another word of advice to Warren would be to limit liquid intake with meals—particularly very hot or very cold liquids. Hot liquids may act as a stimulant to the colon, leading to increased cramps. Excessive liquids with a meal may contribute to the postmeal bloating often experienced with IBS. Furthermore, some researchers believe that excessive liquid may dilute the digestive enzymes, making them less effective. Other pertinent advice is to avoid carbonated liquids—which contribute to bloating—and to avoid gum or mints after meals. Gum and mints frequently lead to swallowing air, which in turn leads to an uncomfortable distension of the intestine—much like blowing up a balloon. Carbonated beverages, gum, and mints may all contribute to increased intestinal gas.

Research has shown that frequent small meals throughout the day may lead to less discomfort than one or two large ones. Eating frequent small meals means that your system is not overburdened at any one time. Just as an automobile performs more efficiently at a constant speed, your personal "food processor" works more smoothly when you avoid sudden starts and stops.

Eating too quickly often leads to overeating, for several reasons. For one, your food will expand in your stomach only as digestive juices are secreted. Haven't we all eaten too quickly, only to experience that uncomfortable, bloated feeling some 30 minutes or so later? In addition, the hormone cholecystokinin, which is released from the duodenum into the bloodstream in response to a meal, goes to the satiety center in the brain, telling you when you've had enough. If you eat too quickly, your body does not have time for this process to occur. As one dietitian proclaimed, "I tell my clients to make love to their food . . . savor each bite."

Whenever possible, make mealtimes a chance to relax. Do not conduct intense business at mealtimes; do not carry on emotionally charged family discussions while trying to eat. Arguing or watching disturbing stories on the news while you're eating may prompt your "food processor" to reject lunch or dinner, leading to acid indigestion. In short, remember that it is often the circumstances surrounding the meal, rather than a specific food, that can worsen digestive symptoms.

CAFFEINE, ALCOHOL, AND NICOTINE

In addition to the act of eating, there are three other common triggers of symptoms. Caffeine, alcohol, and nicotine are often referred to as "social drugs." They are, in fact, drugs in every sense of the word, and yet they are socially accepted—although tobacco use is becoming less socially acceptable as users find themselves increasingly ostracized when they indulge in public. As for alcohol and caffeine use, I believe the best course— whether or not you have a digestive problem—is using only moderate amounts of these substances—if you do not eliminate them altogether.

Many of my patients find it very difficult to give up coffee when I suggest it. "It gets me going," they say. True. For many, caffeine serves to "jump-start" their engines to overcome the inertia of arising. In this regard, caffeine, which stimulates the central nervous system, acts much like an amphetamine, with its energy-boosting characteristics. Unfortunately, over a period of time, humans can develop a tolerance for caffeine, just as they do with other drugs. What this means is that it may later take two or even three cups of coffee or tea in the morning to "get the engine revving." In addition, as the effects from the initial cups of coffee wear off, a withdrawal period ensues—fatigue sets in, and it takes more coffee, tea, or cola, periodically throughout the day, to boost the engine level.

Now I am not trying to spoil any pleasure you may derive from caffeinated beverages. I am simply explaining why it may be most difficult for you to give up caffeine, even though you may conclude that it aggravates your digestive problems.

These inherent difficulties stem from the simple fact that

caffeine—like other drugs—is addicting, and you may well experience an unpleasant period of withdrawal as you reduce or eliminate your consumption. Symptoms of caffeine withdrawal include decreased energy, irritability, and so-called "caffeine-withdrawal headaches."

At this point, you may be asking yourself, "Why, pray tell, should I give up coffee if giving it up will make me feel this bad?" The fact is that your use of caffeine may be making you feel even worse now and you simply don't realize it. Furthermore, after experiencing a brief period of withdrawal symptoms, you will probably find that you feel better and actually have more energy than you did while you were a caffeine "addict."

Many people depend on caffeine to stimulate a bowel movement in the morning, and it may, in fact, help some people who are prone to constipation "keep regular." However, since caffeine is somewhat of a colonic stimulant, it may well exacerbate the crampy abdominal pains and diarrhea experienced by many IBS sufferers. If you rely on caffeine each morning to stimulate a bowel movement, you may find a warm cup of decaffeinated herbal tea works equally well in helping you keep your schedule.

If you are prone to constipation, keep in mind that bowel function is considered to be subject to habit. Therefore, you should allow a period of time at about the same time each day for a bowel movement. Once established, this daily ritual may be more helpful as a colonic stimulant than the morning cup of coffee. Current medical opinion is that those who are very constipated are actually blocking out, or unconsciously ignoring, the urge to have a bowel movement. A popular health adage puts it this way:

When Nature calls, don't try to bluff her,
But haste away without delay, or you will surely suffer.

In addition to intensifying the cramps and diarrhea associated with a spastic colon, caffeine has other adverse effects on the digestive system. It may produce inflammation and even cause ulcers to form in the stomach by stimulating increased secretion of stomach acid. Even decaffeinated coffee, like caffeinated coffee, contains tannic acid, which may aggravate ulcer symptoms. In addition, caffeine relaxes the lower esophageal sphincter (LES), the valve between the esophagus and the stomach. This relaxation sometimes allows acid in the stomach to back up into and burn the esophagus, leading to heartburn or acid indigestion.

As a stimulant, caffeine may also worsen anxiety-related symptoms associated with IBS, such as nervousness and palpitations. Incidentally, if you are a female suffering from painful fibrocystic breasts or premenstrual syndrome (PMS), you should avoid all caffeine. See Chapter 13, "Facts about Coexisting Conditions," for a further discussion of PMS.

Coffee, tea, and many cola drinks contain caffeine. In addition, caffeine is often an ingredient in noncola carbonated beverages and is sometimes used in over-the-counter pain relief medications. Always check the labels for ingredients or contents.

I hope all this evidence will give you reason to eliminate or at least reduce your ingestion of this "social drug."

It may be that small amounts of alcohol have "medicinal properties." After all, it helps you unwind after a stressful day, and alcohol is often found in many cough preparations. However, anyone who has ever experienced a hangover is well acquainted with the consequences of overindulgence. Even drinking what may be considered moderate amounts of alcohol can trigger unpleasant digestive symptoms. Alcohol, like caffeine, may promote inflammation and ulcers in the stomach. IBS sufferers may find beer particularly bothersome, as this carbonated beverage often contributes to belching, bloating, and excessive gas. If you now use alcohol to help you relax, perhaps it will become less necessary as you learn more about stress and relaxation techniques in Chapter 7, "How Emotions Affect the Intestinal Tract." But if you do use alcohol, remember that moderation is the key.

I will spend only a brief time on the adverse health consequences of the last "social drug," nicotine. Most people are aware of the deleterious effects that nicotine, particularly cigarette smoking, has on the body. They know that it causes cancer, emphysema, and heart disease. But did you know that it also causes increased secretion of stomach acid and decreased LES pressure, predisposing smokers to heartburn and peptic ulcer disease? Smokers have increased salivation and swallowing as a result of smoke irritation, and they also experience drying of the mucosa lining of the mouth and throat. The phenomenon of air swallowing (aerophagia) mentioned earlier increases the air in the stomach and the associated bloated feeling often experienced with IBS. If you are a smoker, add these facts to your list of reasons to stop smoking. If your spouse smokes, encourage him or her to stop for your benefit as well as his or her own, since the hazardous effects of secondhand smoke are now well known.

If you sincerely want to stop smoking, read Appendix 6 and seek the advice of your physician.

WHAT TO EAT

You have learned *how* to eat and what common IBS triggers to avoid. The next logical question is, *what* can I eat? Assuming—for the time being—that you have no food sensitivities, or that you are unaware of having any, I recommend the same basic diet for everyone. Food sensitivities are discussed in Chapter 5, "Tracking Down Problem Diet Factors." This "ideal diet" will not only make you less susceptible to IBS but should also help control your weight and give you abundant energy.

You are probably thinking: "This sounds too good to be true. Does this guy believe in the good fairy too?" If you happen to be overweight, you have probably experimented with lots of other diets. An obese patient once told me, "I have lost a thousand pounds over the past fifteen years." Sadly, with dieting, this often happens. Weight is lost only to be regained, then lost again.

Personally, I do not like the word "diet," because it conjures up thoughts of deprivation in the minds of those who have been placed—or have placed themselves—on a diet. Deprivation diets invariably lead to feelings of depression, and depression, in turn, leads to failure. The key, then, is to change your eating habits rather than "going on a diet."

Changing Your Eating Habits

There are only two basic requirements to remember if you want to change your eating habits (or make any lifestyle changes, for that matter). These two basic requirements are *motivation* and *knowledge*.

Pain is a very strong motivational force for many—as an IBS sufferer, this discomfort has obviously motivated you to seek help. You may be further motivated by a desire to lose weight or increase your energy level.

The second requirement—knowledge—provides you with the necessary information to achieve your goal. How much calcium do I need? What vitamins should I take? How can I get more fiber in my diet? These are all questions that my patients frequently ask. Unfortunately, in the area of nutrition, there is an abundance of misinformation. Many patients have told me that the more books they read by so-called nutritional experts, the more confused they become. In addition, whereas current nutritional wisdom places a greater emphasis on increased intake of complex carbohydrates (such as breads, rice, pasta, and beans), these foods were not necessarily emphasized in the past. The point is that recommendations may change as new facts surface.

The Ideal Diet

Now, having said all that, just what is this "ideal diet" that I recommend? Most people are aware that the average North American diet is much too high in sugar, fats, salt, and protein. As discussed in Chapter 5, "Tracking Down Problem Diet Factors," a meal with a high fat content may exacerbate IBS symptoms. Excessive sweets and too much protein also seem to worsen symptoms in many people, at least to the extent that these foods take the place of needed complex carbohydrates in the diet. In addition, excessive salt leads to fluid retention, which may contribute to that "bloated" feeling.

So the "ideal diet" should be high in complex carbohydrates, low in fats (particularly saturated fats and cholesterol), with moderate amounts of protein (see the Glossary for definitions of these terms). Limit your intake of sweets and salt. Sounds simple, doesn't it? Actually, proper nutrition *is* rather simple, but if you are now on the average North American diet, plan to change your eating habits gradually and permanently. You can reduce your intake of sugar, fat, salt, and protein, and learn to relish more healthful alternatives.

This brings up the next natural question. Is it possible to have palatable, appetizing dishes without salt, rich, creamy sauces, and sugar? I say, unequivocally, YES! Realize that butter, salt, and sugar are actually only flavor enhancers. We just got carried away with their use at some point, as in the cliché "if a little is good, more will be even better." The solution is to try to use the smallest amount possible of these substances to complement any dish you are preparing. Instead, experiment with fresh herbs and spices to enhance flavor.

As a native of Louisiana, I grew up with a passion for good food. I enjoy cooking as a hobby and come from a family of excellent cooks. Through the years in our household, we have learned, largely through experimentation, to prepare wholesome and delicious meals with very small quantities of the traditional flavor enhancers. Make a point of experimenting with new foods and new recipes. (See the end of this chapter for two excellent sources of nutritional information.)

FOOD INTOLERANCE OR SENSITIVITIES

By following the advice in the preceding sections, you may very likely notice a complete or substantial improvement in your symptoms. If not, it may be that a certain food or foods contribute to your continued discomfort. (You may discover these foods by using the elimination diet in Chapter 5, "Tracking Down Problem Diet Factors.") Or it may be that your continued IBS symptoms result from your gut's response to emotional stress. The effect of emotions on the gastrointestinal tract is discussed in Chapter 7, "How Emotions Affect the Intestinal Tract." The concept that certain specific foods may produce IBS symptoms has merit, since, after all, your gut is bombarded with a variety of foods throughout the day. In past years, we did not enjoy the variety of foods that are available today. Many people lived in rural areas and raised or grew most of the foods they consumed. It was much easier to trace problem reactions to foods that were eaten rarely—particularly seasonal foods. Prepackaged foods and food additives were much less prevalent then than now. Today it is difficult to discover if chronic symptoms are occurring in reaction to foods eaten daily—or several times a week—or to ingredients that may be "hidden" within preprocessed preparations. The presence of such hidden foods may help explain the increased prevalence of IBS, or spastic colon, in our affluent society.

The consensus among physicians today is that food indeed plays a part in producing IBS symptoms in a proportion of IBS sufferers. However, opinions differ as to the mechanisms, manifestations, and frequency of food allergies. "Allergy" may not be the most precise term to use when describing the majority of patients whose symptoms worsen when they eat certain foods, since allergy in the true sense of the word usually fails to occur.

With a true allergic reaction, a disruptive interaction occurs between the substance to which you are allergic (the allergen) and your body's preformed antibodies. This process sets into motion a series of events that may cause symptoms, such as wheezing, shortness of breath, hives, flushing, skin rash, and occasionally abdominal cramps and diarrhea. Most people's IBS dietary reactions do not involve the interaction of allergens and antibodies.

That is why we often speak of a "food intolerance," or "food sensitivities." It really is largely a matter of semantics. Call it what you will, certain people experience worsening symptoms with certain foods, and the mechanisms underlying these "reactions" differ. An example of the most common food sensitivity will help explain these concepts.

Juanita was an 18-year-old college freshman I saw some six weeks after her first semester of school. She complained of frequent loose bowel movements, crampy abdominal pains, and excessive gas. Her bowel movements were more numerous and bothersome just before exams. While obtaining a detailed history, I learned that Juanita had developed a taste for ice cream because the school cafeteria had an ice cream dispenser. I suggested that she eliminate all dairy products for a trial basis of two weeks. During a follow-up visit, she reported an almost complete resolution of her symptoms, except for occasional diarrhea and cramps preceding "big tests." Juanita's major problem, it turns out, was a sensitivity to dairy products, a so-called "lactose intolerance," although she did seem to have a tendency towards the "spastic colon" variety of IBS when she was placed in a stressful situation.

Lactose Intolerance

Dairy products are the foods most likely to produce or exacerbate symptoms. In fact, I have found many patients to have a pure lactose intolerance without the underlying intestinal disorder seen in IBS.

What happens with lactose intolerance? You may recall from the discussion of digestion that your body produces various enzymes that break down large molecules into smaller molecules, which are more easily absorbed by the intestines. Lactose is a complex sugar molecule found in dairy products. Under ordinary circumstances, lactose is broken down into its constituent simple sugars: glucose and galactose. The enzyme responsible for this reaction is found in cells of the small intestine and is called lactase. For reasons that are unclear, as you grow older your body loses the ability to make the lactase enzyme. If your body is unable to digest and absorb lactose, then this complex molecule remains in the intestines, where it is acted upon by normal intestinal bacteria, leading to symptoms of carbohydrate malabsorption—namely, cramps, gas, bloating, and diarrhea.

Here are some important facts to remember about lactose intolerance:

- It becomes more common as you grow older.
- It is more common in certain ethnic groups—particularly among people with African or Asian origins.
- Since the lactase enzyme is found in the intestinal cells, an infection of the gastrointestinal tract such as "intestinal flu" may damage these same cells and produce a temporary intolerance of dairy products.
- A hydrogen breath test may be used to determine the presence of lactose intolerance. (See Chapter 15, "Common Tests You May Face.")

Does lactose intolerance mean you can never again enjoy dairy products? The answer is no. Fortunately, you may now obtain milk that is treated to be lactose free. You will find that this milk tastes sweeter, since the lactose has already been broken down into its constituent sugars. Alternatively, you can treat milk yourself with over-the-counter lactase enzyme drops to reduce or eliminate its lactase content. Lactase enzyme supplements are also available; when taken with dairy products, these aid in digestion and the absorption of lactose.

If you elect to avoid all dairy products, I strongly recommend that you consider taking a supplement with calcium and vitamin D to prevent later development of osteoporosis, particularly if you are female. There are multiple calcium supplements on the market. It has been recommended that you test whatever brand you buy by placing it in a small cup of vinegar to see if it dissolves, as it should within 5 to 10 minutes. Some calcium supplements are not very well absorbed. Vinegar approximates the acidity of stomach acid, in which calcium supplements should begin to break down for later absorption in the small intestine. The usual recommended intake of calcium is 1000 to 1500 milligrams per day. In North America, approximately 60 percent of the daily intake of calcium is derived from milk and other dairy products. Other sources of calcium include meats, certain fish, and green, leafy vegetables.

Nowadays lactose intolerance is common and easily recognized by most physicians. However, it was not understood until 1965. Before that time, those with pure lactose intolerance would have been lumped together with others considered to have IBS. It may turn out that as our present understanding of IBS increases, we may discover still other enzyme deficiencies that appear to cause IBS symptoms.

Fructose and Sorbitol Reactions

More recently, fructose and sorbitol intolerances have been described. Fructose is a sweetener in many soft drinks (for example, "high-fructose corn syrup"), and sorbitol is a sweetener found in many "sugar-free" or dietetic products. These substances produce effects similar to those seen with lactose intolerance. (See Appendix 4 for a lactose-free diet.)

Other Food Sensitivities

Enzyme deficiencies are only one of the mechanisms by which foods may worsen IBS symptoms. I have mentioned how common triggers such as caffeine and nicotine may lower esophageal sphincter pressures and increase intestinal rhythm. Citrus fruits and juices may also worsen symptoms, presumably by increasing the sugar load and acid load (citric acid) in the intestinal tract.

Certain vegetables—particularly the cruciferous vegetables, such as broccoli, cabbage, cauliflower, and brussels sprouts—are not easily digested by some people unless well cooked or puréed in a soup. This is indeed unfortunate, since the cruciferous vegetables may help reduce the incidence of colon cancer.

The role food additives play in producing IBS symptoms has not yet been completely explored and evaluated. However, the relationship of food additives to other disorders is clear: sulfites have a negative effect on asthma, and monosodium glutamate (MSG) may precipitate migraine headaches. Sulfites are used as a preservative in the processing of wine and beer and in restaurants to maintain the crispness of fruits and vegetables (commonly where salad bars exist). Monosodium glutamate is used as a flavor enhancer in many packaged and frozen foods. Until we understand more about the role of food additives and IBS, you would do well to remember the motto of Boston's Bread & Circus Whole Food Supermarkets and try to eat only "the food, the whole food, and nothing but the food."

SUMMARY

Proper nutrition is essential for those with chronic conditions such as IBS.

Although specific foods may trigger symptoms for some, it can be simply the manner of eating that aggravates IBS symptoms.

It is important to understand the value of a relaxed atmosphere while eating.

Liquids with meals, meals that are too large, the social drugs, enzyme deficiencies, unbalanced nutrition, and modern food additives all contribute to digestive problems.

FURTHER READING

Jane Brody's Good Food Book is a well-researched, comprehensive nutritional guide written by Jane Brody, a health columnist for *The New York Times*.

Cooking Light is published yearly by the publishers of *Southern Living Magazine* and contains a variety of easy-to-prepare, nutritious recipes that are "guided by the premise that good health and good food are synonymous."

5

TRACKING DOWN
PROBLEM DIET FACTORS

By now, you will begin to see the picture: your diet may affect the way you feel, and everyone's digestive system is unique. The diet that is trouble free for you may not be so for someone else.

We all have subtle dietary nuances that make us individuals. How we eat, what we eat, and when we eat may all play a part in intensifying IBS symptoms in susceptible persons. The most common foods thought to induce sensitivities include dairy products, wheat, citrus fruits and fruit juices, chocolate, and eggs. Sweets and meals with a high fat content are troublesome for many people. Suffering from IBS does not necessarily mean you will react negatively to any or all of the above; nor does this list include all foods that have been linked with sensitivities. So how do you track down any special food sensitivities you may have?

THE IMPORTANCE OF USING A DIET DIARY

You must assume an active role if you wish to track down any complicating factors that may contribute to your IBS symptoms, and you must be introspective. A diet diary is the chief tool to

36

help you achieve this goal. All you need is commitment, a pen or pencil, and a notebook.

First, record what you ate and when. You may want to record your diet diary in a notebook and base it on the example below, or you may want to copy and use the sample pages in Appendix 1. Either way, you may follow the instructions for keeping a diet diary in this chapter. When keeping your notebook, be as specific as you can regarding quantities and types of food (including brand names)—remember the hidden ingredients in many preprocessed foods. For example, an entry might read:

> 11:30 a.m.—1 tablespoon of Brand X Chunky Peanut Butter, with 2 tablespoons of Brand X Strawberry Preserves, and 2 slices of Brand X Bread (white).

Such an entry will give you much more valuable information for later analysis than simply writing down:

> Lunch—peanut butter and jelly sandwich

It is also important to record foods in the order you ate them, since you may find you cannot tolerate some foods on an empty stomach, whereas the same foods may be safely eaten with other foods. Don't forget to list all condiments and liquids you consume. For example:

> 1 tablespoon of butter, 2 tablespoons of Brand X Thousand Island Dressing, 12 oz. Brand X Diet Coke.

In addition include the type of day you are having:

> Rushing, late for work, relaxing day at the beach, etc.

Finally, record the type and timing of any symptoms you experience:

8:00 a.m.—Feeling nauseous.
2:30 p.m.—Bloated, excessive gas.

I suggest keeping this type of diary at least two weeks before attempting to determine if there are any patterns. Obviously, the longer you keep your diet diary, the more helpful it will be, particularly if you go out for, say, Chinese food, only once a month. When eating out, make a note of the restaurant you dined in, and inquire about the contents of any sauces, stuffing, or casseroles. I have two patients who can tolerate all types of seafood with the single exception of scallops. They must be careful when ordering stuffed flounder, for example, as scallops may have been used in the stuffing.

Your diet diary will help you become a medical detective, so you may be able to later eliminate or reduce the possible offending agents in your diet. Many of my patients return to me to review their diet diaries, and during this process they are able to determine the specific food groups and circumstances that worsen their symptoms. You may also find that your symptoms are related more to your stress level on a given day than to any specific foods. Or you may discover that on days you skip breakfast and lunch and have a large dinner late in the evening your symptoms are particularly bad. In addition, many overweight patients who take the time to record food intake are surprised by how much they actually eat, and use their diet diary as an aid to reducing calories. Periodically, retest your system to refine and amend the list of foods to which you experience an adverse reaction.

The diet diary is a tool to help you and your doctor analyze and become aware of your daily food habits and choices. It works best if you fill it out immediately after eating or drinking. The diet diary is most helpful when kept daily. If you tend to eat more on weekends or social occasions, make sure to note those days and occasions in the diary.

It is important to record *everything* eaten, including condiments (for example, 1 tablespoon Brand X mayonnaise on sandwich, 1 teaspoon white sugar in coffee) and all beverages, including water (for example, tap water or Brand X bottled water), that you consume.

Record any symptoms you experience and the time they occur. Note the stress level ratings on the sample form (Appendix 1) and circle the appropriate number corresponding to your range of stress levels on that day. List any exercise or physical activity that exceeds your usual activities of daily living. And make sure to take the diet diary with you to your next doctor's appointment.

A More Thorough and Complex Approach: Using an Elimination Diet

The elimination, or exclusion, diet is an alternative and more precise approach to tracking down your food sensitivities. This procedure, though sometimes necessary, is more involved than keeping a diet diary and looking for patterns. And since it could require a restrictive diet for an extended period, during it your body may not receive all the nutrients it requires. Therefore, I recommend the use of an elimination diet only while under the supervision of a physician or nutritionist. Such a diet is not intended to deprive or punish you, but rather to help you gain peace of mind in knowing what foods you can tolerate, and to help you identify those that clearly are problematic.

Basically, the exclusion diet consists of eliminating certain foods from your diet and then gradually reintroducing those food groups and charting your body's reaction. This reintroduction of food groups is called "rechallenging" and is discussed in greater detail later in this chapter.

Fortunately, food intolerance is not very complex in the majority of cases. In isolated instances, however, it may be necessary to sharpen your detective skills if you still suffer symptoms after following the advice so far in this book. For example, suppose you have taken care to eat slowly, chewing food well and in a relaxed atmosphere; you have eliminated caffeine, alcohol, and nicotine; you have modified your present diet to more closely resemble the "ideal diet"; and you have experimented with avoiding such common triggers as dairy products, wheat, fats, and sweets. If you have followed all of these recommendations and are still having problems, then it may become necessary to try an elimination diet. Because diarrhea and gas are more frequently complaints of those with food reactions, if these symptoms persist, an exclusion diet is the best tool for determining whether you have a food intolerance or sensitivity.

As you begin to tackle this difficult problem, do not take the negative approach: "I can eat hardly anything." Rather, emphasize the positive—what you *can* eat! The goal is to determine what foods you can tolerate, and the reward will be the security of knowing there are foods you can enjoy without troublesome symptoms.

Stress as another factor in the development of IBS symptoms is discussed in detail later. Unfortunately, you need to be ever aware of both emotional and physiological stress as a trigger of symptoms so as not to wrongly implicate a particular food. With this idea in mind, you will also realize the importance of periodically retesting certain foods, to see if they must remain on your restricted list. Stress may be one of several factors that make food intolerance seem to be intermittent. Some food intolerances develop over time (for example, lactose intolerance becomes more common with advancing age); others may occur temporarily (for example, after a bout of gastroenteritis or a course of antibiotics).

If you suspect that just a few foods are causing a reaction, you need eliminate only those foods. For example, lactose intolerance is diagnosed by eliminating dairy products from your diet for a specified time. If your symptoms disappear during testing, rechallenge your digestive system at a later date to see if symptoms reappear.

It is best to use the simplest form of the substance when retesting your system. For example, when retesting for dairy product intolerance, drink a glass of milk rather than eating a bowl of ice cream. Ice cream also contains sugar, heavy cream, eggs, and flavorings and additives, all of which may confuse your diagnosis. The issue may actually be more complex than that. Milk consists of three main ingredients: sugar (lactose), protein (casein), and fat. Granted, lactose is the more likely culprit when individuals react negatively to milk. Rarely, we see a true protein "allergy" to casein, and the fat content of milk will bother some, but they can still drink skim milk without difficulty.

As a further example, when retesting for wheat sensitivity, obtain a whole wheat cereal without sugar or additives, rather than whole wheat bread, which may contain other ingredients, such as sugar and yeast. Gluten is a wheat protein found within the wheat kernel. Wheat bran is the outer coating of the wheat kernel. Many people who are intolerant of whole wheat products are reacting to the gluten and may tolerate the wheat bran. Conversely, some people can tolerate refined white flour and react to whole wheat products, suggesting a sensitivity to the outer bran coat of the wheat kernel. I am really not trying to confuse you; I am simply using these examples to point out some of the complexities of food intolerance.

"Aren't there any tests you can perform to determine which foods I am allergic to?" is a question I am frequently asked. Unfortunately, the few tests available are of limited use. Skin tests and the RAST (radioallergosorbent test) will identify those rare individuals with true allergies to certain foods, in which the body has preformed antibodies to a particular food—milk protein or casein, for example. It will not detect the more common food intolerances, such as lactose intolerance, which is the result of enzyme deficiency. From a practical point of view, using an elimination diet remains the most effective way to discover your food intolerances.

To my knowledge, there is no single exclusion diet that is generally accepted and that can be used by everyone following a course for dietary manipulation. In fact, many physicians who treat IBS, or spastic colon, downplay the contribution of food intolerance. This position is defensible, because making common-sense dietary changes and avoiding common, well-established IBS triggers will usually be enough.

Specialists in gastroenterology and those physicians with a special interest in treating IBS generally see the tougher cases, referred to them after the usual therapeutic approaches have failed. For them an exclusion diet may be very useful, unless, of course, the physician suspects emotional or other factors such as adverse reactions to medications, or even a different diagnosis.

A recent study reported that symptoms improved in 48 percent of patients placed on an exclusion diet for three weeks. The patients were chosen for the study because they had not improved with "conventional therapy." However, this study did not address the multiplicity of mechanisms underlying food intolerances.

Foods to avoid when following an elimination diet, together with those foods generally allowed, are listed below. I have compiled this list based on a review of the literature on food intolerance and IBS, as well as my own experience in treating this disorder. Some physicians may think that this list is too restrictive, whereas others may find it incomplete, and I again caution you to use the exclusion diet *only* under the supervision of a physician or registered dietitian.

I advise you to closely adhere to the following points while on the exclusion diet.

RULES FOR FOLLOWING AN ELIMINATION DIET

- Never eat a food that may have caused a life-threatening reaction in the past, even if that food is on the list of allowed foods.
- Exclude any foods from the following "Foods Allowed" list that you have previously identified or suspected as a cause of symptoms.

- When possible, and under the direction of your physician, avoid all nonessential medications, whether prescription or over-the-counter. Otherwise, what you suspect to be a reaction may actually be a side effect caused by the medication.
- Stay on the exclusion diet for a period of two weeks. During this time, eat *only the foods allowed*. If you are not prepared to strictly adhere to the diet, do not waste your time. Any variation will invalidate the results, requiring you to start all over again.
- Read all labels carefully! Many foods or substances on the list to avoid may be hidden in prepackaged or processed food products. Whenever possible, eat fresh, "whole foods" in an unadulterated state. By avoiding prepackaged and processed foods, you may discover if you have any sensitivity to food additives. (See Chapter 9, "Planning for Digestive Security," for a discussion of food labels.)
- Remember that food intolerance or sensitivity is often quantitative as well as qualitative. In other words, small amounts of a certain food "trigger" may not produce negative symptoms, but once the amount exceeds a certain threshold, symptoms will occur. Furthermore, some troublesome foods may only produce negative symptoms when eaten alone and yet are tolerated as part of a meal.
- As you begin, keep a diet diary, as discussed earlier in this chapter. If your symptoms have not improved at all within two weeks, then it is unlikely that food intolerance is a factor, and you should consult your physician regarding other approaches to your treatment. If symptoms improve, you may begin the reintroduction phase of the diet.

Begin your exclusion diet when your life is stable and free of new activities or special stresses. However, be careful not to procrastinate by waiting too long for a stress-free starting date.

FOODS TO AVOID

Milk and dairy products

This includes cheese, margarine, butter, yogurt, ice cream, many pastries, many candies, and any food containing milk or milk products.

Grains

Wheat, corn, oats, barley, and rye. This includes any product made from or containing wheat flour. This also includes any product that contains corn, cornmeal, or corn oil, and products made from oat flour.

Eggs

This includes any of the countless processed foods that contain eggs, such as ice cream, pastries, salad dressings, and pasta.

Citrus fruits

Oranges, lemons, limes, grapefruits, and beverages containing citrus juice. Most common reactions to other types of fruit are rare.

Vegetables

Broccoli, cabbage, brussels sprouts, onions, turnips, and potatoes.

Sweets

All foods with a high content of various sugars (the names of these sugars usually end in "ose"), such as sucrose, glucose, fructose, galactose, lactose and the dietetic sweetener sorbitol, corn syrup, honey, and molasses.

Meats and fish

Cured meats, bacon, sausage and luncheon meats, smoked fish and shellfish.

Caffeine

All coffee (even decaffeinated, since the acid content of coffee is high enough to cause problems). Avoid all caffeine-containing teas, sodas, and chocolate.

Alcohol

All alcoholic beverages. Beer and wine may be especially problematic. Initially, nonalcoholic malt beverages should also be avoided.

Miscellaneous

Spicy foods, fatty foods, fried foods, salty foods, creamy sauces, yeast-containing foods, prepackaged or processed foods containing food additives, and carbonated beverages.

FOODS ALLOWED

Beverages

Tap water, bottled and filtered water (without carbonation), caffeine-free herbal teas, apple juice diluted with water.

Bread and crackers

Only wheat-free and gluten-free bread and crackers, preferably made without yeast or milk products. Try products made with rice flour (rice cakes or rice crackers). Consider baking your own bread using rice flour or flours marked "gluten free," such as arrowroot and tapioca. You may need to visit a health food store to find suitable wheat-free alternatives.

Grains

Rice (preferably brown), puffed-rice cereals, without sugar or additives. Grains such as millet and amaranth may be well tolerated by gluten-sensitive individuals.

Vegetables

All vegetables not included on the "Foods to Avoid" list. Cooked vegetables may be better tolerated (organic produce is preferable where available).

Fruits

All other fruits not included on the "Foods to Avoid" list. Cooked, peeled, or unsprayed fruits may be better tolerated. Excessive amounts of fruits and vegetables may cause gas.

Meats and fish

Of all the meats, chicken and lamb are least likely to cause a problem. Turkey, beef, and pork are allowed. Choose a small portion and a lean cut of meat. Stick with the lighter, less fatty fish with white meat such as halibut, flounder, and sole.

Miscellaneous

Note: Homemade soups and stews made from allowed ingredients are very healthful and nutritious. You can freeze individual serving sizes for later consumption.

RETESTING YOUR SYSTEM

Assuming that your symptoms have improved on the elimination diet, it is now time to determine which of the eliminated foods or food groups may have been causing a problem. It is hoped that there will be enough foods you enjoy on the "Foods Allowed" list to give you a nutritious "emergency diet" to fall back on when symptoms flare. You should always have enough "safe foods" on hand, whether at home or while traveling, to help you through a rough time. Your personal list of foods allowed should grow as you reintroduce and discover the foods you can tolerate from the "Foods to Avoid" list.

There are several important points to bear in mind when retesting food groups:

- The reaction to a particular food may be considerably delayed. Therefore, wait to reintroduce new foods every three days.
- Keep track of what you ate, when you ate it, and your symptoms, if any, in your diet diary.
- Keep your meal patterns consistent, preferably eating several small meals during the day, such as three meals with healthful snacks in between meals.
- Eat adequate amounts, at least two or three servings a day, of the foods to be tested, in their most basic forms. For example, drink lots of milk when testing dairy products, rather than eating ice cream or cheese. If no symptoms occur after three days, you may add this food to your "Foods Allowed" list.
- If you have a negative reaction with reintroduction of a food, put it on the "Foods to Avoid" list. Then wait until you are completely symptom free before resuming testing with another food group.

    Plan to retest, at a later date, those foods that seem to initially cause a problem. If, after several such trials, you find a food consistently causes problems, add that food to your "Foods to Avoid" list.

• Review your findings with your doctor or dietitian to ensure that your list of allowed foods is nutritionally adequate.

I usually recommend initial retesting with dairy products, although the order in which you reintroduce foods from the "Foods to Avoid" list is not important. Many patients have a good idea of whether or not they tolerate dairy products before they even begin the elimination diet. I suggest first trying skim, rather than whole, milk. This will prevent confusing a negative reaction to milk fat (found in whole milk) with symptoms due to lactose intolerance. If you have no reaction to skim milk, you may assume that you do not have lactose intolerance. If the issue still remains unclear, you may wish to try the hydrogen breath test (see Chapter 15, "Common Tests You May Face") to accurately assess whether you have lactose intolerance. Over the next few days, reintroduce 2 percent milk, whole milk, low-fat cheese, and other dairy products.

Next, experiment with the various grains, beginning with wheat. Try a whole wheat cereal, which you may eat with milk, if milk is now on the "Foods Allowed" list. Eat wheat bread if you find that yeast is not a problem. Wheat may take longer to produce adverse effects, so test wheat products for at least four days. Gradually reintroduce other grains, such as corn, oats, and barley.

Next, begin testing with cooked whole eggs, citrus foods, and various vegetables. Remember, cooked vegetables may be better tolerated. If a particular vegetable (say, broccoli) causes no problems when cooked, you may try it raw later.

It is prudent to minimize your intake of alcohol, caffeine, sweets, and fats, even though they may not cause a specific problem related to IBS. As I am sure you are aware, these substances should be used in moderation for various other health reasons.

It is to be hoped that the list of problem foods you will identify will be short. Keep an open mind and a positive outlook, and experiment with new foods that you might add to your list of allowed foods.

SUMMARY

We all have subtle dietary nuances that make us individuals. How we eat, what we eat, and when we eat may all play a part in intensifying IBS symptoms in susceptible persons.

Although there are common foods linked with sensitivities, each person's digestive system is unique.

A diet diary is the chief tool to help you track down your own food sensitivities and reactions. First, you record what you ate and when. Be as specific as you can regarding quantities and types of food. Then record any adverse effects you experience. Eliminate those foods that trigger adverse reactions.

The elimination, or exclusion, diet is an alternative approach to tracking down your food sensitivities. This diet should be used only while under the supervision of a physician or dietitian. Basically, the exclusion diet consists of eliminating certain foods from your diet, then gradually reintroducing those food groups and charting your body's reaction.

With the help of a diet diary, a pattern of reactions may emerge. And if symptoms have not improved at all within two weeks, it is unlikely that food intolerance is a factor. In this case, you should consult your physician regarding other possible treatments. If symptoms improve, foods may be reintroduced as described.

6

DISCOVERING THE VALUE OF HIGH FIBER

For decades, many professionals have advocated an increase in dietary fiber as the cornerstone of IBS treatment. Fiber is the undigested portion of fruits, vegetables, and grains. Although conflicting reports have emerged from time to time regarding the efficacy of fiber in treating IBS, when the sources and quantities of fiber are taken into account, the results are consistently promising. In fact, there has been a resurgence of interest in using dietary fiber for the prevention and treatment of a wide variety of diseases, including diverticulitis, colorectal cancer, chronic constipation, diabetes, and elevated cholesterol.

Is this simply another food fad? Absolutely not! It is easy to understand the resurgence of interest in increased dietary fiber when we realize that in countries where the intake is high, the incidence of all the disorders mentioned above is correspondingly low. In addition, before the 1900s—when people ate whole foods rather than the refined foods of today—these same diseases were much less prevalent.

Chapter 4, "What You Should Know about the Role of Diet," pointed out the importance of increasing your intake of complex carbohydrates (fruits, vegetables, grains). Such a diet, which is high in complex carbohydrates, is also an excellent source of natural dietary fiber.

WHAT DIETARY FIBER DOES

Dietary fiber is not a single food substance. Fiber is a collective term describing a variety of plant substances that are resistant to digestion by gastrointestinal enzymes. During the time fiber-rich substances remain in the intestinal tract, they produce a number of beneficial effects.

From a mechanical standpoint, fiber adds bulk to the stools, thereby actually helping to reduce the intestinal pressure needed to move intestinal contents along. In contrast, a diet high in refined carbohydrates has been stripped of most or all of the naturally occurring fiber. These refined carbohydrates—or so-called "simple sugars"—are almost completely digested and absorbed. What remains in the intestines is only a small amount of residue, creating small, hard stools, which require an increase in intestinal pressure at each bowel movement. The net result may well be constipation and cramps.

From a metabolic standpoint, complex carbohydrates increase energy level, help stabilize blood glucose, and help reduce blood cholesterol. These beneficial metabolic effects explain how high-fiber complex carbohydrates work to prevent diabetes (excess sugar in the blood) and arteriosclerosis (hardening of the arteries). The following examples show how these beneficial effects occur.

The complex carbohydrates found in high-fiber foods must be chemically broken down into smaller molecules before they can be absorbed as simple carbohydrates. This procedure takes time, and calories are actually burned up in the process. This helps to explain complaints of "I am cold all of the time" in those who generally skip breakfast and whose intake of complex carbohydrates is correspondingly low. Eating a breakfast rich in complex carbohydrates is like adding extra wood to the glowing embers of a fire that has been allowed to die down overnight.

The simple carbohydrate glucose is a small molecule and is the major source of the body's energy. When complex carbohydrates are eaten, they slowly break down and are transformed into glucose through a series of metabolic reactions. At the same time, blood glucose gradually rises and falls again. But when you eat something consisting mainly of refined carbohydrates—such as a doughnut made of bleached flour and topped with a sugar glaze—your blood glucose will rise rapidly, and your body will bypass the usual metabolic reactions. This may give you a sudden boost of "quick energy." However, as with many other things in life, you pay a price for this "quick energy," as the body overreacts to this higher-than-normal blood sugar by pouring out insulin from the pancreas in an attempt to decrease the blood glucose. Often the body overshoots, and the extra insulin secreted eventually leads to the symptoms of hypoglycemia or low blood sugar—mainly headache, fatigue, nausea, and nervousness. If you are wondering why the body does not do a better job of regulating such things as blood sugar, it is because your body will work more efficiently if you consume the fuels provided by nature in their original state. After all, have you ever seen a candy bar growing on a tree?

The Different Types of Fiber

Fiber consists of six subtly different substances. Basically, the components of fiber are divided into two groups: those that are soluble in water (pectins, gums and mucilages, and some hemicelluloses), and those that are insoluble in water (lignins, cellulose, and the remainder of the hemicelluloses).

Fruits, vegetables, and grains are not composed exclusively of either soluble or insoluble fibers but contain various amounts of these different compounds. One example of a largely water-insoluble source of fiber is wheat bran, which consists mainly of cellulose and hemicellulose. In contrast, water-soluble fibers have a tendency to retain more water. Some examples of these are bananas and apples, with their high content of pectins. Oat bran, which has received considerable attention recently, is another source of water-soluble fiber.

Water-soluble fibers are also acted upon more than insoluble fibers by bacteria in the colon, through a process known as fermentation. The fermentation process is thought to be important to the formation of an easily passed, moist, bulky stool. Beans, which have a high content of gums, are an excellent source of water-soluble fibers. Unfortunately, as you are probably well aware, beans often give rise to distention and excessive gas. Bloating and gas, in turn, may worsen existing bowel symptoms. The key to increasing dietary fiber, without negative side effects worsening an irritable bowel, is to increase your intake of high-fiber foods gradually. Remember, start low and go slow! Your system will generally adjust over a period of time. Also recall that everyone's digestive tract is a bit different, so trial and error may become necessary to find and eliminate those foods that are most disruptive to your digestive system. For example, I have one patient who tolerates most fresh fruits. However, she has found that plums tend to worsen her symptoms.

The average North American consumes approximately 15 to 20 grams of fiber daily. Most nutritionists recommend twice this amount—30 to 40 grams—as beneficial in preventing those conditions that may result from too little dietary fiber. Some nutritional experts recommend adjusting total fiber intake according to total amount of calories consumed. For example, it may be difficult to consume 30 to 40 grams of fiber if you are on a 1,500-calorie diet for weight control, or if your caloric requirements are low. In these cases, 12 grams per 1,000 calories may be a more appropriate recommendation.

Appendix 5 contains a list of foods high in dietary fiber, which should give you some sense of the fiber content of various fruits, vegetables, and grains. Try to obtain your daily fiber requirement by including a variety of foods from this list in your diet. If you are unable to achieve this goal, perhaps temporarily, because of travel away from home, or chronically, as the result of negative reactions to high-fiber foods, you may be able to complement your diet with one of the many fiber supplements available at drugstores, health food stores and supermarkets. Most of these come in powder form, which, when mixed with the appropriate amount of water, are taken around mealtimes. In this way, the supplement is allowed to mix with the food, helping to provide for soft, formed stools. Psyllium, a water-soluble fiber derived by grinding up seeds from the plantago plant, is the most common ingredient in fiber supplements. It may be found, reasonably priced, in food stores using bulk containers.

I recommend that anyone who is overweight take fiber supplements before mealtimes so that their appetites may be somewhat curbed. Many experts believe that fiber supplements can "normalize" the alternating diarrhea and constipation seen with IBS. During the constipated phase, the water-retaining properties of the fiber allow for a softer stool, whereas during the diarrheal phase, the extra water is absorbed, making the stool firmer. Remember that these supplements contain supplemental fiber; they do not contain the variety of minerals and vitamins found in fruits, vegetables, and grains. Therefore, if you use these products in place of fruits, vegetables, and grains to obtain adequate fiber, check with your doctor regarding the possible need for vitamin and mineral supplements.

SUMMARY

Increased fiber has long been the cornerstone in treating IBS, nervous stomach, or spastic colon.

A diet high in complex carbohydrates is also rich in natural fiber.

The term "fiber" does not describe a single food but rather a variety of plant substances that resist digestion by gastrointestinal enzymes. When these undigested substances remain in the intestinal tract, they produce a variety of beneficial effects. Whereas refined carbohydrates alone may lead to small, hard stools, complex carbohydrates increase energy level, help stabilize blood glucose, and reduce blood cholesterol.

Daily fiber intake can be increased with a variety of foods listed in Appendix 5.

There are supplements available to add desired fiber where necessary.

7

HOW EMOTIONS
AFFECT
THE INTESTINAL TRACT

Earlier chapters described how emotions may lead to physiological responses. Manifestations of this include butterflies in the stomach and nervous diarrhea during periods of increased stress. Blushing in response to an embarrassing situation
is another classic example. This chapter reviews stress, how it
relates to the autonomic nervous system, how stress may lead to
distress, and how you can learn to deal more effectively with
stress.

It is difficult to give a brief, all-inclusive definition of stress,
because the word itself has developed many different connotations. Quite simply, stress may be any stimulus that requires adaptation or change. As things are constantly changing in life, the
way you react physically and emotionally to change determines
how much distress you experience as the result of life's various
stressors.

SOURCES AND TYPES OF STRESS

A social readjustment rating scale has been developed that gives
a relative value to life's various events. The death of a spouse
rates the highest number of points; minor law violations such as

receiving a traffic ticket earn the lowest score. Even events that you may consider positive—such as promotion at work, marriage, and Christmas—are all given relative values on the stress scale. The common denominator is that all of these life events require a degree of adaptability or change.

The same stress that affects one individual minimally may affect another individual with much greater intensity. You may have planned and shopped ahead for Christmas, as you look forward to being with family and friends. Conversely, you may be one who has to rush around at the last minute to find the "perfect" gift for everyone on your holiday list. An individual's personality often dictates whether or not a given degree of stress results in distress.

The classic Type A perfectionistic personalities place undue stress on their systems by making unrealistic demands of themselves. They are often disappointed and depressed when they do not achieve their unrealistic goals. Stress-prone individuals often feel that they are victims of circumstances with no control over their lives or environments—they tend to approach life with a certain degree of negativity and defensiveness.

For sufferers of IBS or "nervous stomach," uncontrolled symptoms may interfere with sexual activity, and this could, in turn, produce marital discord. The resultant heightened tensions may, in turn, worsen IBS symptoms, and so on.

During my residency training, I spent some time moonlighting in the emergency room of a nearby army medical center. I encountered many fresh recruits in their first few weeks of basic training who were experiencing intense abdominal pains. The stress of their new environment, army cuisine, having drill sergeants as surrogate parents, and elimination patterns unaccustomed to military schedules (bowel movements at 0600 hours), had all exacted their toll. The recruits' digestive tracts had essentially shut down. Abdominal X rays revealed colons full of feces, and these usually responded favorably to a few enemas or laxatives.

You can begin to see how abundant the sources of stress are.

As physicians, we must attempt to care for the total individual, recognizing the psychological as well as the physical factors, and understanding that there are life circumstances that will create stress for nearly everyone.

Is all stress, then, bad? No. Actually, under appropriate circumstances, so-called "positive stress" stimulates creativity, facilitates change, and may help you reach peak efficiency. Many people work quite well under pressure and are able to sit back and relax after meeting the challenge. This relaxation response allows them to accumulate the physical and emotional reserves needed to meet the next task. Stress becomes negative when you remain geared up, and you are unable to relax after the challenge. You become like the crew of a warship that remains at full battle stations long after the threat is over. This continual state of arousal sets up a perpetual energy-draining cycle, which causes your health and well-being to suffer.

CHRONIC STRESS

Chronic stress shows itself in different ways in different people: tension headaches, chest discomfort, fatigue, muscle aches, susceptible to infection, and, yes, "nervous stomach" or irritable bowel syndrome. Professionals agree that there is a dynamic interplay between mind and body with any medical condition. With IBS, the symptoms themselves become stressors, and if not dealt with effectively, this stress can feed on itself, worsening your symptoms. Because the gastrointestinal system is closely associated with the autonomic nervous system, it is particularly vulnerable to stress.

A brief review of neurophysiology may clarify how chronic stress adversely affects the body.

The autonomic or automatic nervous system is concerned with functions that ordinarily are not under conscious control, such as heart rate, respiratory rate, and digestion. You do not tell your heart to beat faster or slower; nor do you direct your gastrointestinal tract to digest your food. These functions occur automatically.

The autonomic nervous system is divided into two branches. The sympathetic branch prepares one to meet a threat or challenge by—among other things—increasing heart rate, increasing respiratory rate, and increasing the blood flow to muscles. Various stress hormones, which include adrenaline and cortisol, mediate this so-called "fight or flight" response. The parasympathetic branch, through its major mediator acetylcholine, is concerned with conserving energy. Stimulation of this system results in decreased heart rate, decreased respiration, and increased blood flow to the digestive organs. In this way, your sympathetic and parasympathetic nervous systems ordinarily work like a rheostat to maintain homeostasis or balance appropriate to the given situation.

For example, imagine you have just finished your evening meal and decide to take a relaxing stroll around the neighborhood. Although it is already dark, you are unconcerned because your neighborhood is considered relatively safe. Strolling in a leisurely fashion past a row of bushes, you note they have not been trimmed lately and resolve to bring up this fact at the next neighborhood meeting. Suddenly you hear a rustling among the leaves. A large figure looms out of the darkness, a long shiny object in his right hand as he silently approaches. You are overcome with fear, sensing imminent danger.

Without thinking about it, your sympathetic nervous system is stimulated to prepare you for this threat. Your pupils dilate, you breathe ever faster, you begin salivating (to keep your windpipe from drying out during breathing), and your pulse quickens. Your muscles tense as they receive increased blood flow, which has been shifted away from your digestive organs, and your adrenal and thyroid glands increase their secretion of stored hormones.

Thoughts race through your mind as you contemplate your options: should I run, or should I stand my ground and use the self-defense techniques I learned in Tae kwon do last summer?

You realize your throat is so tight you could not yell for help if you wanted to. Then, as the figure moves into full view in the light afforded by a street lamp, you recognize your neighbor carrying a pair of hedge clippers. "Nice evening for a walk, isn't it?" he declares as he puts out his hand in greeting. "I simply can't seem to find time to trim these hedges during the day, so I thought I'd work on them tonight."

A few moments later you continue your walk. Your sympathetic nervous system begins to wind down, and your parasympathetic system resumes its normal functions, allowing you to relax once again and digest your dinner.

Every week, most of us face stress in our daily lives. When life's daily stresses result in distress, it is usually the result of a prolonged arousal of the sympathetic branch of the autonomic system. This prolonged arousal may lead to fatigue, muscle tension, skin disorders, headaches, and altered digestion. Some people readily admit that emotional stress makes their digestive symptoms worse. Others cannot accept stress as a possible contributing factor to their sense of well-being; they cannot readily identify the stressors in their lives.

The American Digestive Disease Society considers stress a disease. In fact, this may be the best way to view *chronic* stress. You may feel that you have no stressors in your life, that you have a nice family, a good job, and so on. However, for many, chronic stress is an insidious, pervasive problem. It may not be the result of readily identifiable "life events," such as divorce or the death of a loved one. However, illness is a well-known stressor, and as mentioned previously, the increased stress resulting from IBS symptoms will only serve to exacerbate the problem. This is not to say that stress is the root of your symptoms or that it is "all in your head." The symptoms you experience are real and very annoying. To whatever extent you learn to recognize these symptoms of stress, and learn to deal effectively with them, you will be able to exert more control over your autonomic nervous system and help your body function appropriately.

MANAGING STRESS

The first step in learning to manage stress is to identify the stressors in your life. A stressor is anything that causes stress for you. As mentioned, a stressor for one person may not cause much stress in another. It may be difficult for you to pinpoint these stressors. Often subconscious worries or concerns—such as unresolved marital conflicts, financial pressures, or lack of self-confidence—create the most distress. If you are prone to stress, closely examine those attitudes that seem to result in unnecessary stress. Do you make unrealistic demands on yourself? Do you always attempt to control every situation? Do you feel unfulfilled if all of your goals are not met? If you are unable to identify sources of stress, it may be helpful to ask a psychologist to guide you.

We all have stressors in our lives, and how we perceive them and deal with them will determine how much distress we experience. How you relate to the people and events in your life may be a source of chronic stress, if these relationships are not addressed and dealt with appropriately. After identifying the stressors, you must learn to "listen to your body" for the related symptoms: headaches, tension, fatigue, or disordered digestion.

Avoid stressful situations whenever possible. For example, if you hate getting caught in traffic, try leaving for work a little earlier, when the streets are less crowded.

Often, learning to manage your time more effectively is an excellent way to reduce chronic stress. You may find you are wasting a lot of your time and energy running around needlessly working on projects that should be given a much lower priority. I strongly recommend the book *Time Power* by Charles R. Hobbs, or his cassette series, *Your Time and Your Life* (see Further Readings for more information). Hobbs has said that "time management is the act of controlling events" so that you achieve "balance, harmony and appropriateness among the events in your life." Stress often is a result of life's events, and although we cannot control all of the events in our lives, most of us have much more control than we realize. We may learn to focus our energies appropriately and so achieve balance and harmony.

Barbara, a 33-year-old housewife and bookkeeper, works outside the home from 9:00 a.m. to 3:00 p.m., four days a week, doing bookkeeping for a dentist. She visited me complaining mainly of constipation and intermittent abdominal cramps. After obtaining a social history from her, I learned that she was, in every way, a Supermom, Superwife, and Superemployee. But Barbara never took time for herself. She related: "I don't even have time to go to the bathroom."

My "prescription" for Barbara was to schedule time during the week for herself. At first, she expressed guilt about taking this time. However, I pointed out that she really could not continue her present course, because it was damaging her health. After all, that was why she came to my office in the first place. She was doing great things for her children, her husband, and her employer, but she was neglecting to care for herself with the same diligence.

I enlisted the help of Barbara's husband, who wholeheartedly agreed with my suggestions. He described his wife as a person who "could never say no." I learned that financially she had no need to work outside the home as much as she did; the young dentist she worked for had gradually asked her to increase her hours as his practice grew.

Barbara is now job sharing, cutting back to two days a week. At my suggestion, she rises a little earlier each morning—before the children. She uses this time to read, relax, and plan her day. On her last visit, she proudly announced: "My stomach no longer bothers me, and our family life is as good as it ever was." She and her husband now plan at least one night a week to enjoy "dates" together.

I hope this example will help you to see that you can take control of some of the stressors in your life.

RELAXATION TECHNIQUES FOR STRESS

For stressful situations that are unavoidable, there are relaxation techniques that have proved very successful. Stress management consists of first identifying the things in your life that cause you to feel stress. Second, you learn to focus on how you feel under stress. Finally, when you begin to feel stress in the form of distress, you need to be able to relax. When you relax, you will notice a decrease in muscular tension, a slowing of your heart rate, slowing of your respiration rate, and facilitation of the digestive process.

You may already use some relaxation techniques from time to time, such as taking a warm bath, listening to music, working in the garden, or going for a walk. I enjoy reading a good book when I feel the need to relax. However, there are other, more specific relaxation techniques that can be learned and practiced to become an integral part of your daily life. In this way, you can use daily stress reduction as a means of achieving a higher level of health.

As discussed earlier in the description of the sympathetic nervous system, rapid breathing is a response to stress. In contrast, breathing slowly and deeply is an obvious way to neutralize stress. This basic relaxation technique can be performed anywhere and at any time. It is a good idea to practice deep breathing for a few minutes several times during the day, but particularly if you begin to feel tense.

Here's how: Place your hands over your abdomen and feel your stomach expand. Inhale slowly and deeply through your nose. Hold your breath for a second or two, then very slowly exhale through your mouth. Repeat this cycle several times until you feel at ease. Appendix 7 contains a script for making your own relaxation tape.

Another useful relaxation technique involves visual imagery, which is similar to daydreaming. It is best performed while sitting upright in a comfortable chair. Assume a relaxed position, then let your mind take you on a mental vacation. For example, you are lying on a beach and there is beautiful sunshine. You feel the warm rays on your skin, and a cool, gentle breeze. With each breath, your body is invigorated by the clean, fresh air. You hear waves splashing against the shore, and sea gulls calling in the distance.

With practice, you can learn to give yourself well-deserved mental vacations with relative ease. One word of caution: never practice your relaxation techniques in a situation requiring you to be fully alert, such as while driving—or reading this book!

Progressive muscle relaxation is another easily learned relaxation technique. It is most helpful for those who report feeling tense. This technique is best performed in a quiet environment, either sitting or lying down. The basic procedure takes about 15 minutes and consists of alternately contracting and relaxing various muscle groups. In this way, you learn to distinguish between control and relaxation. Begin by contracting the muscles around the eyes, as you would if you were squinting in a sand storm. Hold the tension a few seconds, then relax. Repeat the cycle three times before moving to another group of muscles. By the time you have moved from head to toe, your muscles should be warm and relaxed. Yoga and various martial arts, such as t'ai chi, combine muscular activity and mental relaxation. As one yoga instructor commented to me, "It's like meditation in motion."

Exercise is another excellent means of reducing stress and tension, and physically fit people tend to handle stress more easily than unfit people. The important role of exercise is discussed in Chapter 8, "The Importance of Proper Exercise."

If you lack self-confidence or find it difficult to be assertive, consider taking a self-help course to learn better communication skills. For stressful situations that are unavoidable, there are relaxation techniques that have proved very successful. Always try to maintain a positive approach to life in general. And if you ever find that life's stresses become unbearable, seek professional help. Consult your physician, who may be able to make the appropriate referral, or consult a counseling psychologist. There are also books (see Further Readings) and courses that will help you reduce stress.

Summary

Stress can result from anything that requires adaptation or change.

Stress affects each one of us differently. We often place undue stress on ourselves by making unrealistic demands on ourselves and setting unrealistic goals.

All stress is not bad. Positive stress stimulates creativity, facilitates change, and may help some reach peak efficiency. Stress becomes distress if it remains unrelieved for an extended period of time.

Our gastrointestinal system is closely associated with the autonomic nervous system, which is particularly vulnerable to the effects of prolonged stress.

How you perceive and deal with the stresses in your life helps to determine the amount of distress you experience. A positive self-image, attitude, and lifestyle are essential elements to successfully managing stress.

Stress management techniques *can* be very effective for reducing the negative effects of stress.

8

THE IMPORTANCE
OF PROPER EXERCISE

Often my IBS patients are puzzled when I encourage them to become more physically active, suggesting that this will help improve their digestive symptoms. They ask, "How will exercise help my bowels?"

Skip is a single graduate student. He came for help with classic digestive problems. His symptoms had begun a year before, and they consisted of constipation and crampy abdominal pains, with brief periods of diarrhea. Now, Skip struck me as being an easygoing intellectual type.

During our first interview, I learned that his dietary habits were atrocious. He subsisted on coffee, doughnuts, and fast food. He was almost proud of the fact that he could visit all the area's fast-food vendors and just order "the usual." Overcoming his initial skepticism, Skip began improving his diet and admitted he felt better. He still suffered periods of cramps and constipation but was basically satisfied with his progress. It was at this point that I recommended he increase his physical activity.

Skip offered countless reasons not to increase his activity. He thought the fitness craze was "just another yuppie trend. Besides, I don't have the time. I never liked exercise. I may start when I finish my thesis." And so on.

Finally, after additional inducement, Skip began incorporating some simple exercises into his daily schedule. During a follow-up visit, he commented, "I have not been constipated in months. Every morning I take a brisk walk, and this seems to facilitate a bowel movement." He was very surprised to learn exercise could stimulate bowel activity. It was obvious to me he had never walked a dog.

THE BENEFITS OF EXERCISE

Exercise is one of the elements of a total lifestyle program to help achieve and maintain good health. Exercise helps reduce stress by providing an outlet for aggressive impulses, because stress hormones tend to dissipate during periods of increased physical activity. It makes sense that when your "fight or flight" response is triggered, exercise is an excellent way to neutralize this reaction. Endorphins, naturally occurring morphinelike analgesics, are released after prolonged and continuous exercise. This phenomenon seems to account for the so-called "runners' high." It also explains why some people actually become addicted to exercise, braving all types of undesirable weather to get their fixes.

In addition to helping alleviate digestive symptoms, there are other potential benefits of regular exercise. These include lessening of fatigue by improved physical endurance, increased flexibility, mobility, and strength of the musculoskeletal system, lowered cholesterol and triglyceride levels, and improved posture, appearance, and general self-image. A regular fitness program may save you money in the long run. Exercise can reduce both the need for medication and visits to the doctor about your digestive symptoms, your high blood pressure, or your diabetes. Those who are physically fit find they are less susceptible to injury and disabilities, such as lower back pain, tendonitis, and sprains. Regular exercise will have a positive impact on all aspects of your life.

WHAT TO KNOW BEFORE YOU BEGIN

This chapter provides information about exercise in general and some useful suggestions for finding a program that is right for you. For most people, there is little risk if you begin with less vigorous exercises, gradually increasing your activity level. However, if you are over 30, it is best to have your physician obtain a history and perform a physical exam, especially if you have a pre-existing medical condition. An exercise stress test (an electrocardiogram taken during exercise) may be a good idea, too, depending upon your age, heart disease risk factors, previous level of activity, and other criteria. The exercise stress test is also a helpful tool for your physician or an exercise specialist to use when assessing your most appropriate exercise intensity, based on your maximum attainable heart rate.

In most instances, your body will alert you to potential problems resulting from overdoing it. The old "no pain, no gain" or "do it until it hurts" clichés are dangerous concepts to apply to exercise. If you begin to experience dizziness, palpitations, breathing difficulties, chest pains, or muscle or joint pains, slow down or stop altogether. Chest pains and breathing difficulties are especially worrisome symptoms, as they may be early signs of cardiovascular disease, warranting medical evaluation. Always consult your doctor for advice specific to your particular situation.

You'll find your first challenge is to change your attitude towards a lifestyle that includes regular exercise. We live in a society that emphasizes economy of motion. We use elevators, escalators, shuttle buses, power steering, power brakes, and many other "labor-saving" devices. So begin your attitude adjustment by increasing your caloric expenditure during your normal daily activities. For example, take the stairs rather than the elevator; park farther away and walk instead of looking for the closest parking spot. With these "mini-exercises" you will burn extra calories throughout the day.

CHOOSING THE TYPE OF EXERCISE TO DO

What type of exercise is best for you? There are two basic forms of exercise that contribute to maintaining health. The first type includes those that improve tone and strengthen the musculo-skeletal system. These are stretching exercises, calisthenics, yoga, t'ai chi, and weight training. I personally like to perform some simple stretching exercises for about 20 minutes each morning. "Wake up call" for me is usually the same time each day, so, once established, this routine is easy to keep. I find it a great way to help start the day, and most people can find some time in the morning to exercise, even if it means getting up a little earlier. In addition, you may not need as much sleep as before, as you begin to experience the increased energy from your new exercise program.

Aerobic exercise is the second type of exercise to include in your program. It consists of any prolonged, rhythmical activity that uses major muscle groups. This is the type of exercise you most often hear about. Aerobic exercises require oxygen and lead to improved cardiovascular fitness. Any activity that sufficiently increases heart and respiratory rates may be considered a form of aerobic exercise. Their key requirement is movement from one point to another, and they include jogging, brisk walking, swimming, climbing stairs, and bicycling. Of all aerobic activities, swimming is probably the most nearly ideal: it improves aerobic fitness, while at the same time increasing overall muscle tone, without placing excessive stress on your joints. Exercises that use several muscle groups, such as swimming and using rowing machines, cross-country skiing machines, and stationary bicycles with arm levers, will burn more calories per unit of time than other types of exercise, while also improving the tone and flexibility of both the upper and lower body. You can see how certain types of exercise promote increased cardiovascular as well as increased musculoskeletal fitness.

Walking is an excellent, often underappreciated means of exercise. You may be surprised to learn that you burn just as many calories (approximately 100) by walking a mile as you do jogging a mile. Walking is a less vigorous form of aerobic exercise and is particularly well suited for elderly people, or those just beginning an exercise program. A good pair of walking or jogging shoes is all the equipment required.

My personal bias is that jogging should be reserved for those who pursue it regularly. Occasional vigorous running may lead to musculoskeletal aches and pains (such as knee pain, shinsplints, and bursitis). There is evidence that if you jog regularly, your musculoskeletal system adapts, lessening the possibility of adverse consequences. Again, the key is to start slowly and build up to longer distances and faster times.

It is a good idea to try combining different types of aerobic exercises, something frequently referred to as cross-training. For example, you may choose to walk or swim when weather permits, and work out on a stationary exercise bike indoors when the weather is bad. You may be interested in joining one of the wide variety of exercise classes such as aerobic dance or jazzercize. This is a nice way to obtain support and encouragement and, at the same time, meet new people.

DURATION, FREQUENCY, AND INTENSITY OF EXERCISE

As well as the best types of exercise, there are also the questions of duration (how long), frequency (how often), and intensity (how hard). Most fitness professionals recommend aerobic exercise for a minimum of 20 to 30 minutes, three or four times a week, to achieve and maintain proper cardiovascular fitness. Begin slowly with 5 to 10 minutes of exercise. Progress gradually as you increase, at a rate of 1 to 2 minutes every four or five workout sessions, or as you find you can tolerate the increase. Brief periods of warm-up and cool-down right before and after each session are advisable. During these periods, you should perform the activity at a very low level of intensity, or walk briskly in place for a few minutes.

The recommendations regarding type, duration, and frequency of exercise are relatively straightforward. But how hard should you exercise? Traditionally, the exercise intensity has been based on target heart rate zones, and the target pulse is used to determine the average rate at which you should perform the desired exercise. The target heart rate zone is usually between 60 and 85 percent of the maximum predicted heart rate (MPHR).

To calculate your approximate MPHR, subtract your age from 220. As an example, the MPHR of a 30-year-old person is 220 − 30 = 190. For those in poor shape, or those who primarily want to lose weight, a target pulse rate of 60 to 70 percent of your MPHR would be appropriate. In this case, the target heart rate for our hypothetical 30-year-old would be 114 to 133. If you are in poor physical condition, it may take a while for you to maintain your target pulse for the desired 20 to 30 minutes. Remember, you did not reach your present state of unfitness overnight, so be patient. Keep trying, and eventually you will reach your fitness goal.

Without a pulse meter, it may be cumbersome to check your pulse during exercise. For this reason, the Rate of Perceived Exertion (RPE) Scale has been developed. This is a subjective estimate of exercise intensity and can be closely correlated to target pulse rates. We routinely introduce this concept to people undergoing exercise stress testing to prescribe an appropriate intensity of exercise.

When you achieve your predetermined pulse rate, find out where you are on the scale. There is no correct answer, since each person will have a slightly different perception of how hard he or she is working. The response is usually around the middle of the scale. If you rate yourself as in the range of 4 to 6, this corresponds quite well to an appropriate exercise intensity, regardless of your age or previous activity level. The idea is to get a feeling for the appropriate intensity of exercise. Many find this concept useful when later exercising on their own, thus avoiding the need to monitor pulse rate. Here is a representation of the RPE Scale.

Rate of Perceived Exertion (RPE) Scale

0: None
1: Very, very light
2: Very light
3: Moderate
4: Somewhat hard
5: Hard
6: Harder
7: Very hard
8: Very, very hard
9: Extremely hard
10: Maximum

As your cardiovascular fitness level improves, you will find you are able to exercise more vigorously while still maintaining your previous target pulse rate and level of perceived exertion. Your heart has become more efficient. Wouldn't it be nice if this, in some way, allowed your digestive tract to function more effectively?

Your degree of breathlessness is another gauge of exercise intensity. If you are unable to speak without gasping for breath between each word, you are working too hard. In contrast, if you are able to sing the national anthem without taking a breath, you are proceeding too slowly. You should be able to carry on a conversation that requires you to take a breath every four to five words.

The idea of exercise intensity is often difficult to grasp. Whether you use target pulse rate, level of perceived exertion, or degree of breathlessness, ask yourself at the midpoint of your routine, "Can I continue my present level of exertion for at least

15 to 20 more minutes?" If the answer is no, then you are probably working too hard.

I have counseled many patients who overdo it when beginning an exercise program. The resulting aches and pains only discourage further exercise. If you incorporate regular exercise into your lifestyle, you will, with time, begin to realize all potential benefits. You will be in better physical condition to participate in other recreational activities. In addition, you will be able to live a more active and more healthful life as you grow into your "golden years." I encourage each of you to seek guidance from your physician, an experienced trainer, or various books before launching wholeheartedly into a new lifestyle that includes periodic exercise.

SUMMARY

Exercise is one of the elements of a total lifestyle program to help achieve and maintain good general and digestive health. Although it is not clear how exactly exercise is related to bowel function, exercise seems to help with digestive problems, as it does with most other medical disorders.

Calisthenics, stretching, and weight training are exercises for strengthening the musculoskeletal system.

Aerobic exercises require oxygen and strengthen the cardiovascular system.

In beginning an exercise program, the key is to take it easy, gradually building up to more advanced levels.

Progress can be monitored using pulse rate, the Rate of Perceived Exertion Scale, or breathlessness.

9

PLANNING FOR DIGESTIVE SECURITY

Good planning is the key to digestive health. Most agree that to gain financial independence, you must develop a sound financial plan. In fact, the number of financial planners has skyrocketed in recent years. This trend is driven, in part, by the fact that financial security is a comforting and much-pursued goal. I have begun many of my talks on health with development of this concept. "But," you may argue, "this is a book on digestion. What does it have to do with financial planning?" Well, I have found this concept useful in illustrating two points:

First, a sound, well-conceived plan will increase the likelihood of success in any endeavor.

Second, financial well-being will be of no value if your personal state of health does not allow you to enjoy the fruits of your labor.

I have watched patients achieve the pinnacle of success only to have a stroke or heart attack remind them that along the way they neglected to give their bodies proper attention. Granted, spastic colon/nervous stomach/ibs is not a life-threatening condition such as a stroke or heart attack, but negligence will result in troublesome symptoms. The stress arising from uncontrolled symptoms of ibs will only compound other medical problems. I have found that the threat of a future disease is less a motivating factor than the immediate benefits many IBS sufferers obtain from dietary changes. This chapter will help you develop a structured approach to eating and meal planning. And once developed, this plan can be continually refined to help you enjoy a full life.

USING A NUTRITION PLANNER

The suggestions in this chapter should steer you onto the right track and motivate you to absorb new information as you expand your knowledge of proper nutrition and diet. Consider using a dietitian as your personal "nutrition planner" during your quest to obtain digestive health. The dietitians I have worked with have been most helpful in assisting my patients identify their specific food intolerances, develop healthful meal plans (which ultimately benefit the entire family), perform dietary analysis to ensure that all nutritional requirements are met (particularly if you are on a restricted diet), and serve as personal tutors, advisers, and sources of encouragement.

It has always struck me as odd that people will spend hundreds of dollars on prepackaged diets for weight reduction, or for body building, and yet be reluctant to invest a fraction of that amount in individualized counseling with a professional dietitian. (And I find it difficult to understand why they think nutrition in a can is more appealing than eating whole foods.)

There are lots of "nutrition experts" out there, and I suggest you shop carefully for your personal nutrition planner. Ask your friends, your doctor, or others whose opinions you value, for their names. Contact them to see if they are willing to meet with you for a get-acquainted visit. At this time, they will most likely outline their approach to proper diet and nutrition. Most dietitians will request that you keep a record of your food intake. This helps them determine your present dietary habits and discover your food preferences. They may also enter this information into a special dietary computer program for a detailed analysis of your intake of fat, carbohydrates, protein, vitamins, and minerals.

The food intake record serves as a base from which the dietitian can make recommendations for dietary modifications. As previously mentioned, these records are also useful in helping to determine food intolerance.

Some dietitians accompany their clients on a grocery store field trip as part of the program. This is a great place both to talk about and learn about food—much better than a classroom. In addition, the clients learn to read package labels. Understanding these labels is a simple task and an essential part of comprehensive nutritional education. Label reading is explored later in this chapter.

There are a multitude of benefits to a well-structured nutritional plan besides the obvious one of lessened digestive symptoms. For many, weight control is a continual concern, and particularly as we age, those extra pounds seem to sneak up on us. Eating right can help control weight, and a well-balanced diet will also increase your energy level, enhance your self-image, and even help prevent disease and sickness in the future.

In an earlier chapter, you learned to play detective and identify some foods that are bothersome to you. I hope that your list of food sensitivities is not too long or too restrictive. Ideally, the sufferer will be able to consume, with minimal modification, what everyone else in the family eats. And often, when the family diet is modified to accommodate the sufferer, the changes will ultimately benefit all. Always remember that you can return to your baseline diet as needed when you suffer a flare-up of digestive symptoms.

When You Visit a Grocery Store

Living near a grocery store is a mixed blessing. It is certainly convenient when you need to pick up something you forgot or must replenish an item you unexpectedly deplete. However, this convenience makes carefully planned shopping excursions less likely. Many of my patients are from rural eastern Colorado, and I sense that their trips to town for groceries are very well planned. If they happen to omit an item, well, they usually make do. In addition, a last-minute trip to the store for a critical ingredient of your dinner recipe is an added source of stress and a waste of your valuable time.

By now you may begin to sense that the recommendations in this book are all interrelated. Proper meal planning is another way to help reduce stress while following a proper diet, and this combination of proper diet and stress reduction will, in turn, lessen digestive symptoms.

The first step in planning your grocery shopping is to list those items you need. Now, if you are like me, you may need to tie a string around your finger to remember the list. Ideally, you should keep a continual list as you notice you are running out of staples such as milk or bread. Encourage your entire family to use this list, adding those special items they need, or they note are in short supply. Conduct a periodic inventory to identify items not on the list. It is a good idea to maintain a complete list of items you frequently use as a reminder of what to check during your inventory. If you are out of a regularly used item, rather than just low, you may not have a nearly empty container to remind you, but your master list will.

The next step is to prepare a basic menu for the week, or for at least until the next trip to the grocery store. Then add to your list the special ingredients you need for each selected recipe. Now your grocery list should be complete. You may want to arrange the list into various food groups, such as produce, dairy products, and bakery items, to help you save even more time in the store. Saving time in the store will allow you extra time to prepare dinner or simply relax.

Attempt to grocery shop when you are feeling well. The sight and smell of food may make you nauseous or uncomfortable if you must shop while your symptoms are heightened. Avoid shopping when hungry because you may then tend to overbuy. Stick to the list, but take advantage of seasonal availability or "good buys" on items you know you will use. Whenever possible, buy fresh or unsprayed foods; their nutritional value is greater than that of frozen or canned foods. Organic produce is preferable where available.

Try to arrange your grocery trip for a time when the store is not likely to be crowded. This saves additional time, since you will not have to wait in long checkout lines or battle crowded aisles.

READING FOOD LABELS

An intelligent consumer will learn to read food labels, which provide information on the content and nutritional value of food products. The Food and Drug Administration (FDA) in the United States and the Department of Consumer and Corporate Affairs in Canada have set standards for such labeling, although the nutritional information is often incomplete.

If you are on a lactose- or gluten-restricted diet, be aware that these items will not usually be listed on labels as separate ingredients. You need to know that all milk or milk solids contain lactose, and that ingredients derived from wheat, rye, barley, or oats will contain gluten. Some manufacturers may choose to label a product as lactose free or gluten free if it is specially designed for persons with either intolerance.

The list of ingredients must include any artificial flavorings, colorings, or preservatives. A product without any of these ingredients may be labeled as having no additives. Although a product may be labeled as having no preservatives, the same product may contain artificial flavorings and colorings as long as there are no chemical preservatives. Detectable amounts of sulfites must be listed in the ingredient list, because sulfites have been shown to worsen asthma in susceptible individuals. I have not yet seen scientific reports that sulfites worsen IBS, but I have found patients who believe this to be a trigger for digestive problems.

Foods on the ingredient list must be listed on the label in order of their predominance by weight. For example, if sugar is the first listed ingredient (or high on the list), this means the product's sugar content is high. If sugar appears much later or lower down the label listing of ingredients, it is less likely to be a major ingredient. Whereas this listing gives the rank order, it does not tell what percentage of the product each ingredient actually constitutes. If you are attempting to limit sweets in your diet, for example, to decrease gas and bloating, avoid any ingredient that ends in "ose," such as glucose, fructose, sucrose, lactose, and galactose. All of these so-called "simple sugars" may be fermented by colonic bacteria, increasing gas production.

Be wary. Some producers will "split" an ingredient. Instead of using sugar as the only sweetener in a product, they will add honey, corn syrup, or molasses. This puts the sugar content lower on the list, when, in fact, the total content of sugar or sweeteners is high.

LABELING TERMS

The following is a list of terms and definitions imposed by federal regulation to describe various food products. This list may be helpful as you attempt to decrease your intake of fat, sodium, or calories:

U.S.
Extra Lean   Less than 5 percent fat.
Lean or *Low Fat*   Less than 10 percent fat.
Lite, Leaner, or *Lower Fat*   At least 25 percent less fat than similar products.
Sodium Free   Fewer than 5 mg per serving.
Very Low Sodium   Fewer than 35 mg per serving.
Low Sodium   Fewer than 140 mg per serving.

Reduced Sodium   At least a 75 percent reduction compared with the usual content of the food.

Unsalted   No salt added during processing.

Low Calorie   No more than 40 calories per serving, or no more than 0.4 calories per gram.

Reduced Calorie   Minimum of 1/3 fewer calories when compared with usual product.

Canada

Fat Free   Less than 0.1 g fat per 100 g serving.

Low Fat or *Light*   Less than 3 g fat per serving.

Reduced in Fat   More than a 25 percent reduction compared with similar products.

Salt Free   Less than 5 mg per 100 g serving.

Low Sodium, Low in Sodium, or *Light in Salt*   Less than 40 mg sodium per 100 g serving (50 mg sodium/100 g for cheddar cheese, and 80 mg for meat, poultry, and fish). At least a 50 percent reduction in sodium.

No Salt Added or *Unsalted*   No sodium added, and no ingredient contributes a significant amount of sodium.

Reduced Sodium   At least a 25 percent reduction in salt.

Low Calorie, Light in Calories, or *Low in Energy*   A 50 percent reduction in calories. No more than 15 calories per average serving, and 30 calories per reasonable daily intake.

Reduced in Calories, Lower in Calories   More than 25 percent reduction in energy.

Calorie Reduced, Light in Calories   A 50 percent reduction compared with the usual content of the food.

Foods advertised for their nutritional properties, such as "low-fat" or "low-calorie" products, and foods that have been enriched or fortified, such as breakfast cereals, are required by law to have nutritional labels. Other products may voluntarily carry nutritional information on their labels. In both cases, the label must list the total number of calories and the number of grams of protein, carbohydrate, and fat per serving. There are approximately 9 calories in every gram of fat, and 4 calories per gram of carbohydrate or protein. Remember this relationship and you can easily calculate the percentage of fat calories contained within a product. For example, a cup of whole milk contains 150 calories with:

8 grams of protein
11 grams of carbohydrates
8 grams of fat

By multiplying grams of fat by calories per gram (8 grams x 9 calories per gram), we get 72 calories; almost half of the 150 total calories in a cup of milk is derived from fat. This means a cup of skim milk, which contains no fat, has approximately 78 calories (150 − 72). You can see the tremendous decrease in calories, particularly fat calories, you achieve by switching from whole milk (approximately 3.5 percent milk fat) to skim milk.

Nutrition labels in the United States must also include the percentage of the U.S. Recommended Daily Allowances (U.S. RDA) for eight nutrients: protein, calcium, iron, vitamin A, vitamin C, thiamine, riboflavin, and niacin. A listing of other nutrients, such as vitamin D, may be included but is not required. In Canada, nutrient labels are not mandatory, but where they are used, fat, protein, energy, and carbohydrate levels must be listed. However, manufacturers are not required to state levels of vitamins or mineral nutrients, such as iron or zinc.

PREPARING A WEEKLY MENU

Ideally, food preparation begins shortly after your return from shopping. Resealable plastic bags, airtight plastic containers, and recycled glass jars are an invaluable aid for keeping foods fresh and saving leftovers. You may wish to rinse and chop vegetables at this time and store them for later use. Lettuce that is washed, drained, and placed in an airtight container will last longer and is ready for use at any time. If simply tossed into the refrigerator, lettuce—and other vegetables—will often wilt within a few days.

The fact is, you are much more likely to eat salads and fresh vegetables if they are already washed and ready for consumption.

This is also a good time to skin and debone chicken or to filet fish for later use. This will save you time later on, since much of the preliminary work for using these ingredients in a meal will already have been done. Some experts suggest that when you prepare foods in advance, they lose nutrients and freshness. I believe that if this preparation is carried out properly, the loss—if any—will be minimal. The following suggestions will help you enjoy tasty, home-cooked, nutritious meals with a minimum of stress.

Use discarded leafy tops of vegetables and chicken bones for making stock. The more fresh foods you actually prepare from scratch, the less likely you are to encounter the troublesome ingredients found in prepackaged foods.

It is more efficient and economical to prepare larger quantities of certain foods—which you can easily refrigerate or freeze for later use—than preparing each meal from scratch. This way, you have homemade "TV dinners" whenever you lack the time or desire to cook. Some items, such as soups, stews, spaghetti sauce, and casseroles, actually seem to taste better as leftovers. If you are not sure whether you will be using an item within a few days, store it in the freezer rather than allowing it to deteriorate in the refrigerator. Label all containers and include the date. Always throw out any food that may have spoiled. Do not feed it to the dog unless you are prepared to eat it yourself. (Why make Fido sick?)

A New Way of Eating Reduces Stress

Bret was a single executive who hated to cook. He actually felt uncomfortable in the kitchen, and the sum total of his experience in the culinary arts consisted of proficient use of the microwave and toaster. His specialty was microwave popcorn. He knew the precise temperature setting and timing to make a perfect batch.

As Bret advanced within the corporate structure, his stress level increased, and it was at this time that he was referred to me. After reviewing his food intake record, I realized that his diet was a major contributor to his symptoms. But I also felt certain he would be unable to change his dietary habits without some help. Fortunately, the dietitian recommended to him worked with a cook who would not only grocery shop for clients but would actually prepare meals in the home for future consumption.

At first, Bret was unreceptive to the idea of having a personal cook twice weekly; he thought it would be far too costly. He agreed, however, to try it briefly, and the result was a dramatic improvement in his symptoms. He remarked, during a later visit with me, that he felt he was actually saving money because he was brown-bagging it at lunchtime and eating out less. His personalized lunches and dinners were comparable in cost to the frozen dinners he had been buying at the store. Brown-bagging is a sensible, cost-efficient way to control the quantity and content of the food you eat while enjoying home-cooked meals when you are out.

Americans consume more than one-third of their meals outside the home. Given this information, it is encouraging that more restaurants are developing health-conscious menu items. In the next section, there are some preventive health hints for dining away from home.

EATING OUTSIDE THE HOME

Diane called our office one morning seeking advice for intense abdominal cramps and diarrhea. I had not spoken to her in some months, and asked what she thought had triggered this latest episode. Apparently, she had attended a dinner party at a friend's home the previous evening. She was famished when she arrived because she had skipped lunch to run errands and to take one of her children to a doctor. When the host offered wine with cheese and crackers as starters, she could not resist. The appetizer served only to whet her appetite, and when the homemade lasagna arrived, she attacked her plate.

Diane knew she had a low tolerance for lactose-containing foods; had she remembered her lactase enzyme supplements, perhaps she might not have been in her present predicament. She also recalled, the next day, that alcohol, particularly wine, had caused problems in the past. Although she had declined at first, her host insisted she try "a taste." He was right; the wine hit the spot, and after the first glass, she found it even more difficult to decline a refill.

This story suggests several important points. First, that you should give as much thought and preparation to the meals you will eat out as to those you eat at home. Depending on the situation, ask what will be served. Tell the host or hostess ahead of time that you have a digestive disorder (you need not go into any more detail) and that your doctor has suggested you restrict consumption of certain foods. In most instances, your hosts will be able to modify your serving (for example, giving you less gravy, sauce, or cheese) or provide a suitable alternative. At least they will be less likely to insist that you try the wine, rich desserts, or espresso if they know ahead of time that you must exercise dietary discretion. You will end up feeling better and also be more convincing if, for example, you compliment the chef but actually eat only half a portion.

In addition, Diane could have saved herself a lot of discomfort had she remembered her lactase enzyme supplements.

She broke another important rule by arriving at the dinner party hungry. That is not to say she should have eaten a complete meal just before leaving; however, she would have been less inclined to overindulge had she not skipped lunch, or had she eaten a light snack before leaving home. I cannot overemphasize the importance of frequent small meals to help control digestive symptoms.

Alcohol, particularly on an empty stomach, can cause havoc in the digestive tract of an IBS sufferer. It is always a good idea, whether or not you have IBS, to eat a light meal or snack before a cocktail party. This is especially true if you plan to consume alcohol. You will find the alcohol less bothersome, and you will be less likely to overeat. The combination of alcohol and rich hors d'oeuvres does not constitute an ideal meal, and yet if you do not eat something ahead of time, it could very well be your meal for the evening.

Finally, as difficult as it may be at times, be assertive. If you accept and eat a restricted food, *you* are the one who will pay later. I realize that this will often tax your willpower to the limit, especially when what is offered looks and smells really delicious. You do not want to offend the hostess, and she really has persisted in her request that you "at least try it." As one patient remarked to me, "I get in these situations where my taste buds outvote my stomach."

Dining in a restaurant can still be a pleasurable experience, although I do encounter patients who worry about eating out because "I never know if or how I will react to the food." In contrast to a dinner party, you do have a little more choice when you are eating out. Seek out restaurants that offer healthful dishes. Unfortunately, although there are no entrées prepared especially with the IBS sufferer in mind, many report that they find "heart-smart," low-cholesterol, low-sodium dishes quite palatable and without negative reactions. These dishes are generally lighter, and the decreased fat content is less likely to cause problems. Do not be afraid to inquire about the use of additives. For example, ask about the use of MSG, particularly if you are planning to dine in an oriental restaurant. Often, it can be omitted on request.

Avoid fried foods. Request that salad dressings, gravies, and sauces be served on the side. This allows you to control the amount you use, and you may find the dishes delicious without these accompaniments. You do not need the extra calories anyway. Since sweets are a common trigger, do not order dessert until after a meal. You may find you have had enough without one. If you really crave something sweet, order some fresh fruit, or share a dessert with someone else.

TIPS FOR TRAVELING

Many experienced travelers are aware that airlines will provide special meals at no extra cost and that the meal service is not a take-it-or-leave-it proposition. But you must plan ahead and notify the airline at least 24 hours in advance (or tell your travel agent when purchasing the tickets), and request one of their listed special meals. The selections are somewhat limited, but they include a low-calorie, a low-fat, a low-sodium, and a vegetarian meal. These alternatives, although still airline food, are lighter and usually easier to digest than the standard meal.

At your hotel, take advantage of room service if it is provided. In some of the nicer hotels, this is a relaxing way to enjoy an elegant meal in the privacy of your room.

Travel across time zones can often result in jet lag. Rapid transit through time belts, particularly international travel, may lead to fatigue, headaches, and mental clouding. Psychological adjustments may occur quickly, but your physiological functions, such as digestion, kidney performance, hormonal regulation, and the sleep/wake cycle, may take longer to conform to the new schedule. This change is often coupled with a change in diet as you encounter rich, unfamiliar foods during travel. If you are not careful, this may throw your bowels into rebellion. Attempt to stick with your diet and with familiar foods as much as possible when on the road. Take along some "safe" snacks and fiber supplements to use as needed to regularize bowel movements. If possible, plan to arrive at your destination a day early to allow some time for rest and to begin the adjustment process. You may begin preparation for rhythm disturbances in advance by retiring one hour earlier for each hour to be lost going east, or one hour later for each hour to be gained when traveling west. Strive to maintain your regular exercise program. If you are staying in a hotel, choose one with health club facilities.

If you are a frequent international traveler, you may want to become a member of the International Association for Medical Assistance to Travelers (IAMAT). Although it is unlikely that your IBS symptoms will necessitate a visit to a foreign doctor or hospital, IAMAT may provide valuable assistance if a more serious illness occurs while you are away from home. IAMAT provides a list of English-speaking medical personnel around the world. In addition, it can supply information about climate, sanitary conditions, immunization requirements, malarial risk, and advisable clothing. IAMAT's four-page "Traveler Clinical Record" can be used to list your personal medical information. There is no charge for membership in IAMAT. To obtain information, write IAMAT at 417 Center Street, Lewiston, NY 14092, or phone (716) 754-4883.

Other Travel Tips

- Eat a light meal before departure.
- Place an emergency provisions kit in your carry-on luggage. Include such things as herbal tea, individual serving-size boxes of cereal, healthful snacks, lactase enzyme supplements, fiber supplements, and prescribed medications.
- Avoid eating gas-producing foods before departure.
- Wear loose-fitting, comfortable clothing.
- Avoid alcohol before and during a flight.

SUMMARY

Planning is the key to digestive health.

Consider using a carefully chosen dietitian as your personal nutrition planner during your quest to obtain digestive health.

Most dietitians will request that you keep a food intake record to serve as a base from which to make recommendations for dietary modifications.

Eating right can help control weight and will also increase your energy level, enhance your self-image, and even help prevent disease and sickness in the future.

Plan and organize your visit to the grocery store in advance to avoid stress and to ensure that you accomplish what you set out to do.

Learn to read food labels.

The more fresh foods you actually prepare from scratch, the less likely you are to encounter the troublesome ingredients found in prepackaged foods.

Give as much thought and preparation to meals outside the home as for those consumed inside. Tell a host or hostess ahead of time that you have a digestive disorder and that your doctor has suggested you restrict your consumption of certain foods.

When dining out, always remember any medications such as lactase enzyme, and request the lighter dishes.

Learn to be assertive. If you accept a restricted food item, *you* are the one who will pay later.

Take special care when traveling to keep to your diet and avoid needless stress.

10

ADDITIONAL TIPS

FOR

TREATING SYMPTOMS

The symptoms of IBS are often intermittent and unpredictable. By now, though, you will have begun to realize that there is no single treatment, trick, or "cure" for the disorder. Many people improve dramatically with dietary and lifestyle changes, and with stress reduction. However, they may have one or two lingering symptoms that become a constant or recurring source of aggravation.

DEALING WITH LINGERING SYMPTOMS

Luc is a 37-year-old real estate professional, working in a crowded real estate office. In many ways, Luc was a classic IBS patient. He had suffered from crampy abdominal pain and irregular bowel movements. He also complained of belching, bloating, and excessive gas. After I had concluded that we were dealing with IBS, I outlined a program of specific treatment recommendations. He responded well to the treatment plan but continued to experience gas.

"Doc," he confided, "I pass enough gas in an afternoon to fill a hot-air balloon. It's embarrassing and uncomfortable, and I can't always control it. I'm afraid that if you can't help me with this problem, my coworkers may see to it that I'm exiled to a deserted island." Then with a grin he added, "It's a good thing it's a nonsmoking office, because there are times it would definitely be inadvisable to light up."

In order of importance, the goals of IBS therapy consist of regularizing the bowel movements and relieving abdominal pain. If you are able to develop a consistent pattern of bowel movements that are neither too hard nor too soft, the abdominal pain will often, in turn, be relieved. Your other symptoms, such as bloating and gas, will also improve once you establish regular, consistent bowel movements. As you know, the pain of an IBS attack is usually relieved by a bowel movement, and that bloated feeling is lessened if you are not constipated.

Luc simply got carried away with the recommendation of increased dietary fiber. As many do, he thought that if some fiber is good, more will be better. After this was brought to his attention, he decreased his daily intake of fiber and has continued to do well.

INCREASING DIETARY FIBER

As outlined in a previous chapter, gradually increasing dietary fiber is an excellent way to regularize bowel movements. Fiber is the undigested portion of complex carbohydrates (grains, fruits, vegetables, beans), which remains in the intestinal tract to exert a beneficial effect. Fiber will add bulk to the stool, making a hard stool softer and a soft stool more firm. Fiber supplements may be added to your diet if you cannot maintain an adequate fiber intake by increasing the amount of complex carbohydrate you eat.

If you do take fiber supplements, be sure to take them around mealtime so that they can mix well with the food. For some reason, many people get into a habit of taking their fiber supplements at night, just before retiring. This is not the best time, and you may end up with a hard stool lodged in the bowel and a gelatinous mass (the fiber) attempting to push it out. If you take the fiber supplement at mealtime, it will mix with the food, providing for a consistent, moist, bulky stool.

"How often should I have a bowel movement?" is a question I am frequently asked. Most medical authorities contend that "normal" bowel function varies between three bowel movements a week and three bowel movements a day. These estimates imply that if you have more than three bowel movements a day, you have diarrhea, and if you have fewer than three a week, you are constipated. However, this so-called "normal" range has been established on the observation that the majority of people in the western world fall between these two extremes. Realize that what is "normal" for you may not be an optimal frequency of bowel movements for someone else. Furthermore, the frequency of your bowel movements may not be as important as the consistency of the stool. You may have a daily bowel movement that is very hard and difficult to pass, suggesting constipation. Conversely, you may have rather infrequent bowel movements that are loose and watery when they occur, suggesting diarrhea.

Although regular bowel movements are important in helping to relieve IBS symptoms, it is also important not to become insistent on this fact. The fact that you do not have a bowel movement does not necessarily point to a problem unless you experience pain, discomfort, and bloating *because* you have not had a bowel movement.

LIFESTYLE FACTORS THAT CONTRIBUTE TO SYMPTOMS

There are several likely explanations for the apparent increase in IBS and other bowel problems in recent years. I propose what I have come to refer to as the outhouse theory. Persons living in rural areas in the past ate a much more balanced, wholesome diet than we tend to eat today in our urbanized, fast-paced society. In addition, in the days before modern rest rooms, the outhouse was the temple of elimination. Many of my older patients who grew up during this era become quite distressed when there is a change in their "regularity" (a valid concern, since this may be a warning signal of colon cancer). These patients tell me that for as long as they can remember, they have had regular bowel movements. They recall scheduled early-morning treks to the outhouse to relieve themselves, before they left the house to start their day.

In today's society, we take for granted the fact that toilets are readily accessible. There is no need to plan a certain time for elimination. ("I will go when I get the urge, whether at home, at work, or in a public facility.") This approach leads to a problem with timing. It may not be convenient for you to go when the need arises, since you may be in an important business meeting or stuck in traffic. And after "holding it" for a period of time, the urge will often lessen to the point where you no longer feel the need. This both conscious and subconscious blocking of impulses from the rectum may ultimately lead to constipation. You may later experience an uncomfortable "crampy" feeling, and then, when you have to go, you *have* to go!

How to Prevent Constipation

You can begin to see that one of the most important ways to avoid constipation is to establish a consistent time for elimination. This is what I refer to as "adult toilet training." For most, the best time is after breakfast. The fact is, meals stimulate the gastrocolic reflex and may facilitate a bowel movement after, for example, a bowl of cereal. As food enters the stomach, a series of events that facilitate digestion is set into motion. The hormone cholescystokinin is released; in addition to stimulating gallbladder contractions, it also stimulates colon contractions—leading to defecation. This hormone is believed to mediate the gastro (stomach)-colic (colon) reflex.

Many patients tell me they are not hungry early in the morning. This is no doubt true, as their systems have been conditioned to skip breakfast, much as an infant may be conditioned to feed on a regular schedule. Perhaps you are the type of person who likes to sleep as long as possible. Since you know it takes exactly 24 minutes to commute to your job, you set the alarm for 7:12 a.m. so that you can be dressed and out of the house by 7:34 a.m. This leaves you precisely 2 minutes to spare before beginning work at 8:00 a.m. And breakfast consists of coffee and doughnuts in the office during your first break at 10:15 a.m.

Why not try taking a break when you first arise? Set the alarm for 6:45 a.m. and use the extra time to eat a balanced, wholesome breakfast at home and to have a bowel movement. This will help relieve your stress level too, since rushing to work tends to set the pace for the remainder of your day.

What about enemas? It is true that an occasional enema may be an effective way to stimulate a bowel movement "from below." Like laxative abuse, the abuse or overuse of enemas may cause problems in the long run, because your rectum can become dependent upon this procedure. Colonics should also be used with caution. "High colonics" are colon-cleansing treatments. This age-old technique uses large volumes of fluids to wash out or cleanse the colon, with the intent of purging the colon of toxins that may have built up. Outbreaks of parasitic infections have been reported in facilities where this technique was used. I have had patients referred to me who have previously undergone this procedure, and they found it to be of dubious benefit.

TIPS FOR PREVENTING CONSTIPATION

- Increase dietary fiber.
- Establish a routine time and place for elimination.
- Allow adequate time for a bowel movement.
- Regular exercise may help prevent constipation.
- Do not habitually use laxatives. (Fiber supplements, however, are not laxatives in the true sense of the word and may be safely used.)
- If you *do* take laxatives (whether prescription or over-the-

counter), use them only for a short period of time, and only under direction of a physician.

HOW TO PREVENT DIARRHEA

Increasing dietary fiber or adding fiber supplements to your diet, in addition to alleviating constipation, can also lessen the discomfort associated with diarrhea. If you suffer from IBS and have a tendency towards diarrhea, look closely for triggers. I find that "diarrhea predominant" IBS patients will have food intolerance or allergies more frequently than their "constipation predominant" counterparts. A study published in the journal *GUT* suggests that food intolerances are more common in patients who first complain of flatus (gas). The most common foods to trigger an episode include dairy products, chocolate, eggs, and wheat products. Nuts, tea, coffee, citrus fruits, and potatoes have also been implicated. Please refer to Chapter 4, "What You Should Know about the Role of Diet," for a more detailed explanation of dietary triggers. Remember that the mechanisms underlying food intolerance are complex, and do not be too quick to eliminate certain foods from your diet without first consulting a physician. Too often, I have seen patients who have placed themselves needlessly on very restrictive diets as a result of inconclusive analysis. In these cases further investigation revealed that the list of foods that may be causing a problem is much shorter than was previously suspected.

Emotional stress is a frequent cause of so-called "nervous diarrhea." If stress triggers diarrhea in your case, please refer to Chapter 7, "How Emotions Affect the Intestinal Tract." Learn, practice, and experiment with different stress reduction techniques to alleviate stress-induced diarrhea. If these measures fail, your doctor may recommend various medications to treat symptomatic diarrhea. These medications are most useful on a short-term, as-needed basis, such as when you are traveling, or where bathrooms are not readily accessible. Take care to not overdo it, or you will end up constipated. Keep in mind that peppermint is an antispasmodic, which may also help the diarrhea and associated cramps. I have many patients who find caffeine-free peppermint tea very calming to the gut.

How to Prevent Abdominal Pain

Your stress reduction techniques and peppermint tea can also be helpful when you are experiencing abdominal pain and cramps. Try relaxing when the urge to defecate or expel gas occurs; this could alleviate symptoms.

Some of my patients find a brisk walk helps to reduce the spasms, and this might also facilitate the passage of gas. Others have said that a warm bath seems to help.

Try focusing your attention on something—anything—other than the pain. With time, the painful spasms will usually pass. Only if all these measures have failed, try taking the antispasmodic medication your doctor may have prescribed.

How to Prevent Excessive Gas

If you have a problem with gas, you need not feel alone. "Gas" is probably the most common of the gastrointestinal complaints. The production and passage of gas is a normal physiologic function, although many consider it socially unacceptable. The source of many a joke, it can be an embarrassing, uncomfortable problem.

The symptoms of excessive gas may consist of belching (eructation), bloating, abdominal pain, and passing gas from the colon (flatus). How is excessive gas defined? Well, believe it or not, the technology is available to measure daily gas production, and studies have been done. The data seem to suggest that IBS sufferers do not produce excessive amounts of gas in comparison with people without IBS. Rather, IBS patients are more sensitive to normal amounts of gas present in the intestinal tract.

The majority of gas in the intestinal tract comes from swallowed air. Also, anything that increases the production of saliva will contribute to increased air swallowing (aerophagia). Part of the "fight or flight" stress response is increased salivation, and nervous tension may therefore be a factor. Cigarette smoking and the use of gum and mints also increases salivation and air swallowing. Thus, the ingestion of carbonated beverages contributes to intestinal gas. Perhaps you recall the time you quickly downed a pop or beer. You felt bloated, and may have felt better after you burped. If the gas does not exit upwards, it will eventually find its way out the other direction. Air swallowing may lead to excessive accumulation of gas in the stomach, which may produce a bloated feeling and pain in the upper abdomen. Belching often makes this condition better.

A word of caution is in order here. There is a difference between a spontaneous belch and a forced belch. A spontaneous belch occurs when air trapped in the stomach escapes through the esophagus, resulting in lessened pressure and decreased bloating. Having observed this, many people attempt to make themselves belch when they feel bloated. However, it has been shown that forced belching is accomplished by actually swallowing air and then belching it back up. More often than not, more air is swallowed than is brought back up by forced belching. The net effect is one of worsening symptoms, since a perpetual cycle develops in which more air accumulates in the stomach. Some people drink carbonated beverages to facilitate belching and relieve the bloated feeling. This practice may also ultimately worsen the symptoms associated with air swallowing.

Air in the stomach that is not eructated will pass along with the chyme into the small intestine, then the large intestine, and eventually out of the rectum as flatus. Along this route, pockets of air may become trapped, producing bloating and "gas pains."

As air rises, it will have the tendency to accumulate in the uppermost areas of the intestine. Two such areas are the upper right colon (hepatic flexure) and the upper left colon (splenic flexure).

Some people have a predisposition to the trapping of air in one or the other area, producing bloating and pain, referred to as either the hepatic or splenic flexure syndrome. The more common splenic flexure syndrome may produce pain that radiates from the left upper abdomen to the left shoulder area.

The discomfort of gas pains may mimic a heart attack. Since heart disease is much more common than splenic flexure syndrome, be sure to consult your physician if you experience this type of discomfort.

In addition to swallowed air, the digestion and fermentation of certain foods will produce intestinal gas. Complex carbohydrates, particularly those with a high water-soluble fiber content, such as beans, are the greatest gas producers. There does seem to be individual variation in how much gas is produced with certain foods. This variation may be related to varying degrees of carbohydrate malabsorption, such as that seen with lactose intolerance. Lactose intolerance is not an all-or-none phenomenon. There seems to be a certain threshold above which the lactose load exceeds the body's ability to break down the lactose. A half cup of milk may be tolerated, whereas a whole cup of milk will produce gas in the same person. You may need to do some detective work to determine what foods may be contributing to excessive gas in your case. Your diet diary would be a helpful tool for this endeavor.

TIPS FOR DECREASING INTESTINAL GAS

- At mealtime, eat slowly and chew your food well in a relaxed environment.
- Avoid excessive liquids at mealtime. Do not "wash down" your food.

- Avoid carbonated beverages.
- Avoid using chewing gum, mints, and tobacco products, which all increase air swallowing.
- Try to determine which foods in your diet are easily digested.
- If you are in the process of adding fiber to your diet, do so slowly, allowing your intestinal tract time to adjust.
- Wear comfortable, loose clothing.

SUMMARY

IBS symptoms are intermittent, and there is no single treatment or cure.

The goals of therapy include regularizing bowel function and relieving pain.

Fiber supplements, a consistent time for elimination, and avoiding the stress of tight schedules all help regulate bowel function.

Emotional stress can trigger "nervous diarrhea."

"Gas" is the most common gastrointestinal complaint, and IBS sufferers seem to be more sensitive to normal amounts of gas.

Certain dietary and lifestyle changes can help minimize gas problems.

11

IMPORTANT FACTS
ABOUT MEDICATIONS

The majority of IBS sufferers will need no medications if they follow the advice in the preceding chapters. I have found medications most helpful only when other avenues proved insufficient, or when used temporarily to relieve specific symptoms. Unfortunately, a number of people think there is a "pill for every ill." They would always rather take medication than attempt to achieve relief by changing their diets or other aspects of their lifestyles.

Although some medications seem to relieve certain aspects of IBS, they are no substitute for a concerted effort to gain self-control through proper diet, stress reduction, and exercise. This chapter gives a brief overview of those classes of medications that are most frequently used to treat IBS. Common trade names are given in alphabetical order in Appendix 3.

Because, as mentioned previously, IBS is not a single disorder, there is no single medication to alleviate all symptoms in every patient with this diagnosis. Similarly, there is no medication that will "cure" IBS. However, some people do undergo a spontaneous remission of symptoms, and others find medications helpful to temporarily relieve particular symptoms.

Your physician can analyze your situation to ascertain which, if any, medications may be most helpful. Just as there are many ways to establish the diagnosis of IBS, each physician may prefer certain medications as a result of personal experience. Also, remember that what works for Aunt Millie may not work for you.

WHAT YOU SHOULD KNOW ABOUT MEDICATIONS

If medications are prescribed for you, make certain you fully understand:

- What is the purpose of the medication?
- How does this medication work?
- Is it habit forming?
- When should I take this medication?
- Should I take it all the time, or only when I have symptoms?
- What might happen if I suddenly stop taking the medication?
- What are the common side effects?
- What are the effects of long-term use?

I mention "common side effects," as it is not practical or worthwhile to list all the possible side effects of a medication. Your doctor will be able to tell you which fairly frequent side effects should concern you. If, however, you begin taking a medication and all does not seem as it should be, check with your physician to see if you are experiencing an unusual side effect.

It is *most* important to check with your physician before taking medication prescribed by another practitioner or purchased over the counter. In this way, you minimize the potential for harmful drug interactions. Be particularly careful with alcohol. It is a common drug that may interact with a variety of medicines, usually causing excessive drowsiness, and impairing ability to drive and to safely operate hazardous equipment.

Just as some people are anxious for medication to resolve their problems, others would rather avoid drugs under any circumstances. I attempt to respect both ends of this spectrum. With this in mind, here are some observations I have made over the past few years about IBS medication.

NATURAL REMEDIES FOR IBS

There are a couple of "natural" remedies that have proved to be of variable benefit. These include peppermint oil and ginger root, both of which may usually be obtained in capsules at a health food store. Peppermint oil, which is also sold in liquid form, seems to help decrease painful intestinal cramps by relaxing the smooth muscle in the intestinal wall. Some of my patients find peppermint tea (caffeine free, of course) helpful for the same symptoms.

I also consider the psyllium seed bulk-forming fiber substances to be "natural" remedies or dietary supplements. Psyllium, which contains water-soluble fiber, is obtained by grinding the seeds of the plantago plant. There are commercially produced products that contain no sugar or additives. Shop around at stores that sell these products in bulk food containers for the most economical product that works for you. (See the chapter on fiber for a more detailed discussion of dietary fiber, and Appendix 3 for an annotated list of medications.)

MEDICATIONS USED TO TREAT IBS

The major symptoms of IBS are abdominal pain and altered bowel habits. The goals of drug therapy are, therefore, to alleviate the pain and regularize the bowel movements. Often, if the bowel movements become more regular through dietary changes or use of fiber supplements, the pain is lessened.

A word about the use of medications during pregnancy is in order. A medication intended for the mother may have adverse effects on the developing fetus. Although the list of drugs that definitely cause fetal abnormalities is relatively short, information regarding the absolute safety of a medication is seldom available. For this reason, I would rather not recommend any medication to a pregnant woman. If you are pregnant or think you may be, check with your physician about the risk and benefits of drug therapy.

Antispasmodics

The first and probably the most commonly used class of medications includes the antispasmodics. These medications are intended to prevent painful intestinal smooth-muscle spasms. The most common side effects of the antispasmodics include dry mouth, blurred vision, dizziness, difficulty emptying the bladder, and constipation. If you experience dry mouth, remember, you may well aggravate your symptoms by using gum or mints or drinking excessive liquids at mealtimes in an effort to combat this side effect. The constipation occasionally experienced with the use of antispasmodics may actually prove beneficial in diarrhea-prone patients. For a constipation-prone patient, I prefer to use antispasmodics only after the bowel movements have been regularized through the use of a bulking agent to increase dietary fiber. Antispasmodics may not be necessary after constipation is corrected, and if needed for occasional cramps, they will be less likely to cause constipation if the bowel movements are more regular to begin with.

Non-Narcotic Opioids

Under certain circumstances, the so-called "non-narcotic opioids" may be prescribed to treat troublesome diarrhea, especially "nervous diarrhea," which may occur on the first day of a new job or on a backpacking trip or another outing where frequent bowel movements may be most inconvenient. These agents achieve their results by decreasing peristaltic activity of the intestinal tract. Their side effects may include drowsiness and constipation.

Antidepressants

Antidepressants have also occasionally been used for IBS. The rationale for using these medications is based on studies suggesting that many patients with IBS are judged to be depressed. Now, whether depression is a cause of IBS or merely appears in association with IBS is not known. In other words, does depression lead to IBS, or do patients become depressed because they suffer from IBS? At any rate, these antidepressants are effective as part of a total treatment plan for some patients with IBS. These same medications are very useful in patients with fibromyalgia syndrome (FMS) as well as IBS.

The side effects of these medications are similar to those of the antispasmodics. They include dry mouth, blurred vision, dizziness, difficulty emptying the bladder, and constipation. (For a list of side effects for each drug discussed in this chapter, see Appendix 3.)

Tranquilizers

Since emotional stress may precipitate IBS symptoms, the anti-anxiety or so-called "minor tranquilizers," are often prescribed to treat this aspect of the disorder. I advise patients to develop coping skills, and to practice such self-help techniques as relaxation training, rather than relying on a particular medication to deal with life's stresses.

However, these agents may be helpful for brief use during periods of significant anxiety. Used daily on a long-term basis, these medications can cause a pattern of physical and psychological addiction to develop. As well as their being habit-forming, other potential problems include oversedation, particularly if taken with alcohol. Multidrug combinations, consisting of an antispasmodic and an anti-anxiety agent, have been widely used for treatment of IBS.

Other Drugs

Medical practitioners have also recommended other drugs for use in IBS. Here is a brief outline of a few that have been used or are being considered for possible benefit.

Metoclopramide is a medication that promotes emptying of the stomach and helps prevent heartburn. It may be useful for treating bloating after meals for some people, if other causes of bloating, such as gallbladder disease, have been ruled out.

The so-called "H$_2$ blockers" are designed to decrease acid secretion by the stomach and thereby promote healing of peptic ulcers. These medications are sometimes used for IBS patients with upper abdominal burning pains, where there is no evidence from endoscopy or upper gastrointestinal X rays demonstrating definite ulcer disease. These pains, which may or may not occur with IBS, are often referred to as nonulcer dyspepsia.

Nitroglycerin preparations, which are traditionally used to treat the chest pains associated with angina, are helpful in treating esophageal spasms and *proctalgia fugax* (painful spasms of the rectum).

Beta blockers and calcium channel blockers are other traditional heart medications, which are being investigated for possible benefit in controlling the abnormal intestinal tract movement in IBS.

A group of medications known as bile-acid sequestrants—which are most useful in treating elevated blood cholesterol—is sometimes helpful in treating those with diarrhea-predominant IBS.

Simethicone is the active ingredient found in a variety of over-the-counter products. It is designed to relieve gaseous distention. Although simethicone is very safe, the evidence suggesting benefit has not been overwhelming. Preparations containing activated charcoal (which is an adsorbent) have shown some possible benefit in adsorbing gastrointestinal gas, thereby aiding patients who complain of excessive flatulence.

Lactulose is a synthetic sugar, which may be useful for

chronic constipation if fiber additives prove ineffective. This agent is held to be relatively safe for long-term use.

This chapter has focused on the pharmacologic treatment of IBS. I have discussed the most commonly used classes of medications as well as other medications that may be of possible benefit. The intent of this chapter has been to give you some insight into the rationale of drug therapy and to help you realize that drug therapy is aimed at treating specific aspects of the disorder. Realize that pharmacologic treatment of any disorder must be individualized by your physician, based on a multitude of factors.

SUMMARY

Medications are sometimes recommended by your physician to treat specific symptoms as needed.

Your physician will prescribe the medications you may need.

Know the facts about your medication: how it works; how and when to take it; common side effects.

There are "natural medications," with rare side effects, that may work well for some symptoms.

It is most important that pharmacologic treatment of any symptoms be individualized by your physician.

12

FOR "SIGNIFICANT OTHERS," ABOUT THE IMPORTANCE OF SUPPORT

IBS can affect all aspects of an individual's life, and as is true for many chronic and recurring medical conditions, the consequences of this disorder will naturally affect all those close to an IBS sufferer. Living in harmony takes understanding.

For example, you're traveling down the freeway to visit Aunt Sarah. Your "significant other," the person you share life with, politely requests that you take the next exit and find a rest room, and you do not. The next request may not be quite so polite, because IBS turns normally compelling desires into urgent ones. As one patient remarked to me, "I don't need the *next* bathroom; I need the *last* one!"

IBS is one of those disorders employees are unlikely to report, simply because employees are embarrassed to blame absenteeism or tardiness on their bowels. One case illustrates this point. A supervisor directed a sympathetic inquiry to my office, wanting to know why one of her subordinates was getting so many "viruses." Could that worker have AIDS? I politely pointed out that I was not at liberty to discuss a patient's medical problem, but I did mention to my patient that I had received a call from her supervisor.

I suggested she level with her boss and tell her that she suffers from the most common gastrointestinal affliction, one that has been estimated to affect up to 22 percent of the population. As it turned out, the supervisor admitted that she, too, suffered similar symptoms from time to time.

This chapter is devoted to "significant others" in the hope that they will develop an understanding of the many manifestations of IBS. If you are in this role, you will learn a little about the disorder, how it can affect your relationship, what you can expect through treatment, and what your significant other may be doing to try to cope with the problem. Through a better understanding, you may be able to develop the support necessary to see your significant other through an IBS attack and to adjust your lifestyle to ease symptoms.

GROUND RULES FOR A HARMONIOUS RELATIONSHIP

First, it is important to discuss and negotiate mutual expectations with all the parties concerned. These expectations can be about such issues as domestic chores, sexual relations, or even such simple matters as how often you will make rest room stops while on a trip. Working out these aspects of a relationship in advance, with participation from all concerned family members, is an important step in building any relationship, even without the added impact of IBS. Such a cooperative effort becomes even more important when one family member suffers from a chronic disorder like IBS. Once you have negotiated expectations in your relationship, make an effort to adhere to them, regardless of the increase or decrease in symptoms on a given day.

Next, be aware that support is a feeling and not necessarily a set of activities. As the significant other of an IBS sufferer, you may need to set limits on the kinds of actions that are required and requested in your relationship. Sometimes an IBS partner will not be aware of being emotionally supported and will seek some action or another from you to affirm your support. In this event, tell the IBS sufferer about your supportive feelings.

Finally, monitor your own level of comfort with the disorder and your level of sympathy with the IBS sufferer. If you find yourself feeling angry or unconcerned about your significant other's disorder, or should you feel entrapped by the illness, you may seek professional help from a therapist experienced in working with family issues and chronic illnesses.

Ideally, you will feel sympathy with what IBS demands of the sufferer. At the same time, you should feel comfortable in expressing your own needs, and content to not constantly demonstrate your care through overt action. Negotiate expectations with your significant other assertively and flexibly, and then follow through consistently.

WHAT IS IBS?

Along with establishing harmony in your relationship, you need to know more about IBS, and how your significant other can attempt to cope with it.

IBS (irritable bowel syndrome), or spastic colon, is the most common gastrointestinal affliction in North America today, so your significant other is certainly not alone. The hallmark of IBS is abdominal pain associated with an altered pattern of bowel movements. Think back to a time when you have suffered the symptoms of a gastrointestinal virus. (One the medical profession refers to technically as the "green apple quick-step," also known as the "trots," or the "runs.") You had cramps with their resultant pain, and the embarrassment from diarrhea was also quite unpleasant. This may be true for your significant other as well.

Others may experience the abdominal pain accompanied by constipation, and still others may have bowel movements that alternate between diarrhea and constipation, and that are never "regular" or "normal."

These are the symptoms that IBS sufferers experience—either constantly or sporadically.

What triggers these symptoms?

There are a number of things that can trigger these unpleasant, often embarrassing symptoms. Two of the most frequent triggers are diet and emotionally stressful situations. It is most helpful to consider them both when helping to ease your significant other through an IBS attack.

People with IBS are often sensitive to certain foods. For example, it would be unwise for you to insist that your significant other sample the chocolate mousse your boss's wife prepared if she says she would rather not. She knows from past experience there will be a price to pay. Simply let her explain, "I'm sorry, but I react to chocolate," and let it go at that. Put this way, I doubt that any hostess would press the matter. After all, no one wants a guest to suffer a bad reaction in his or her house.

In addition, your understanding and sensitivity to what your significant other is going through can help defuse a potentially emotionally stressful situation. Often the primary consideration on the mind of IBS sufferers, whether at a formal dinner, a party, or a backyard barbecue, is "Where is the bathroom?" because they never know when the need will be urgent.

It is best to be sympathetic without making IBS the focus of your lives. Doing so, although well intentioned, will only serve to focus all thought on the problem. Most will agree that if you suffer from a toothache but can find something else to occupy your mind, the pain seems less.

I experienced this at firsthand when my wife and I went through a Lamaze birth preparation class. The instructor had me apply a firm, steady pressure to my wife's upper thigh to the point that she indicated it was painful and asked me to stop.

We then repeated this while she was practicing the highly focused breathing techniques she had learned in the class. It was obvious to both of us that her tolerance to pain increased as long as her mind was focused on the breathing rather than on the painful pressure I was applying. (In fact, if you have been trained as a Lamaze "coach," you may be able to help talk your significant other through a series of intense cramps.)

Under most circumstances, however, it would be preferable

for the sufferer to discuss her symptoms with her doctor, or to try to work things out on her own. Doing so helps her gain a sense of control over the problem. And after all, you may not always be there to offer support.

It has been suggested that recurrent abdominal pain in some children may be the result of a learned or conditioned response to stressful situations. The special attention and treats they receive "to make them feel better" may actually serve to perpetuate the problem. It is felt that these very same children could grow up to develop IBS as adults. This is not to say that their pain is not real or that they are attempting to get attention. However, their symptoms may be magnified when they are allowed to become a recurring central issue. The evidence does suggest that your significant other should receive your love and attention not only when she is not feeling well but also, and most importantly, on those occasions when all seems to be going right. Relish and nurture your relationship on the good days.

As a physician, I encounter many types of spousal relationships, from the one who "couldn't care less" to the one who is constantly concerned, almost to a fault. The first type considers another's problem to be just that: *their* problem, and only a means to get attention from time to time. They are clearly not concerned.

The other extreme is the one from whom I often receive calls: "Why can't something be done? Surely there are more tests. Surely there is some medication to relieve the suffering!" To these, I have to explain that there are certain limitations in the practice of medicine, even today. There is no "quick fix" or cure, and further expensive, often uncomfortable tests will serve no useful purpose. I would suppose this same person inquires every day: "How are you feeling today? Is your stomach bothering you?" The most helpful and appreciated approach lies somewhere between these two. The most important tactic is one of informed, concerned understanding.

From time to time, I have advised some of my patients to seek marriage or family counseling. I sense faulty lines of communication, that IBS or other illness is only one aspect of disturbed family relationships. I sense sometimes the existence of hidden anger or resentment, as in the remark, "We can't even plan a trip because of her bowels... " The response to my suggestion to seek counseling is often surprise or denial: "There is absolutely nothing wrong with our marriage. If we could just get a handle on this spastic colon... "

The fact is, counseling would probably enhance most relationships. I know of too few perfect marriages, and crisis intervention seems to be a North American way of life. My advice: do not wait until the relationship is on the rocks and you are ready to see an attorney to seek professional guidance. In fact, I would like to see family counseling referred to as "family workshops" or "family seminars" to help overcome the stigma attached to it. "Jane and I are attending family workshops" sounds so much more positive than "Jane and I are in counseling."

To emphasize it once more, IBS affects many aspects of marital life, not the least of which is enjoyment of sex. Studies have shown that for many women with IBS, uncomfortable intercourse is a frequent complaint. Patients have related to me: "Who wants to have sex when you're feeling gassy and bloated?" "For years, my husband thought I was having headaches... " And we have yet to learn the impact of the emotional stress such situations foster. If this seems to be a problem area, a professional sex therapist may be able to offer some helpful suggestions.

WHAT CHANGES CAN BE EXPECTED WITH TREATMENT

Since IBS is considered to be a functional disorder, that is, one without a single specific cause, we must treat the symptoms. I have seen relief in those who make significant changes in diet, who exercise, and who practice stress avoidance and stress management techniques.

You may see your significant other keeping a diet diary to re-

cord foods eaten, with reactions to certain foods or food combinations. You may notice changes in social habits like avoiding
coffee, tea, alcohol, or cigarettes. Just because your significant
other suddenly gives up the 5:00 p.m. cocktail with you does not
necessarily indicate a flaw in your relationship. It could very
well be an attempt to discover which factors will exacerbate the
symptoms. And some changes in the timing of meals and where
they are eaten may also occur.

Be ready to see more fiber appear in the daily diet, along with
some changes in the weekly menu, as your significant other
works to produce relief from her IBS symptoms.

Your significant other may begin a program of daily exercises, too. These may be serving a twofold purpose: helping to
improve the body's overall condition and assisting in stress relief.
If you have been accustomed to "couch potatoing" after a heavy
meal in the evening, you may also be called on to make some social adjustments.

WHAT YOU CAN HOPE FOR

Although there is no "cure" for IBS, you can still hope for control. Diet, exercise, stress reduction, and moderation in daily living all play a significant role in this. I have found that many of
my patients respond favorably to a combination of treatments.
And they have begun to rediscover for themselves the normal
daily and social activities that may have been difficult or impossible before. What you can hope for, then, is a return to some
sort of "normalcy," where the activities and events you once
shared can be yours again, without the constant stigma of
"Where's the bathroom?"

In conclusion, I recommend that you be sympathetic and responsive to your significant other's needs during an attack. However, in your daily relationship, do not make spontaneous sympathetic inquiries, or dwell on the subject. When he does feel the

need to let you know what he is going through from time to time, be ready to listen.

SUMMARY

IBS affects all areas of an individual's life, including family and significant others.

IBS is characterized by abdominal pain, associated with an altered pattern of bowel movement, which may create a sense of urgency.

Diet and stress may both trigger symptoms.

Counseling may assist in opening faulty lines of communication and fostering understanding as a couple.

You may see some significant changes in diet and lifestyle.

A return to some sense of "normalcy" and to previous activities is possible with proper management of IBS.

13

FACTS ABOUT
COEXISTING CONDITIONS

IBS, PMS, FMS—sounds a little like some sort of alphabet soup, doesn't it?

Helen, who works as a grocery store cashier, is a good example of someone with this combination of problems. On her first visit, she proclaimed, "I feel like a hypochondriac." She said she had been having problems with her bowels for most of her life. The cramps and diarrhea usually worsened, however, 7 to 10 days before the onset of her menstrual flow. She suspected, after reading a magazine article, that she had PMS (premenstrual syndrome). In addition to her bowel complaints, she experienced mood swings, breast tenderness, and fluid retention during the premenstrual phase. Over the past few years, she had come to accept these symptoms as her fate. Only after she began to experience extreme fatigue and generalized aches did she decide to seek medical attention.

After preliminary evaluation, I determined that Helen had developed, over the preceding 12 months, symptoms consistent with the diagnosis of FMS, (fibromyalgia syndrome), in addition to her symptoms of IBS and PMS. FMS, previously referred to as fibrositis, is a common disorder affecting an estimated 3 to 6 million people in the United States.

Both PMS and FMS are common. FMS, like IBS, occurs more

frequently in women than in men, and of course PMS occurs only in women (although some women contend that men go through similar cyclic changes). It is uncommon for all three disorders to be present and create a significant problem in one person, as they did with Helen. It is not uncommon, however, for two of these three problems to coexist.

PMS

Up to 90 percent of women admit to having some form of premenstrual discomfort. The majority of these women experience mild symptoms that do not interfere with normal daily activities. The lifestyle and dietary changes recommended to treat PMS are similar to those recommended to control IBS symptoms, so if you suffer from both problems, you should be able to improve both conditions simultaneously by following the guidelines in this book.

Symptoms of PMS

The symptoms of PMS vary greatly among individuals. In addition, the number and magnitude of symptoms associated with PMS may vary with each cycle or at different stages of life for each person. Although the symptoms of PMS could well fill a text, these are the more common, generally accepted symptoms: mood swings (anxiety, depression), irritability and headache, breast swelling and tenderness, menstrual cramps, fluid retention, fatigue, and cravings for certain foods (especially sweets).

The hallmark of the disorder is the occurrence of these symptoms 10 to 14 days before the onset of the menstrual flow—hence the name premenstrual syndrome. Studies show that the number of psychiatric admissions, accidents, and suicide attempts among women increases during the premenstrual phase. This phenomenon indicates that mood changes can be quite severe.

Many IBS patients report worsening IBS symptoms in their

premenstrual phase. These symptoms may be the result of hormonal changes that occur during the menstrual cycle, or they might occur as the result of eating salty foods, sweets, and other foods that PMS sufferers tend to crave.

A study recently reported in *Gastroenterology* found that 34 percent of 233 planned parenthood clients who denied symptoms of IBS reported that menstruation was associated with one or more bowel symptoms. IBS patients from the gastroenterology clinic were significantly more likely to experience worsening bowel symptoms, especially increased gas, during menses. It appears that bowel dysfunction increases during the menstrual flow in PMS patients with and without established IBS.

Diagnosis and Treatment of PMS

Although PMS was described more than 50 years ago, there is no general consensus as to the cause or treatment. Nor is there a specific test to diagnose PMS. As with IBS, the diagnosis is suggested by the patient's history, and the physical exam and any tests are used to exclude other disorders, such as endometriosis and ovarian cysts.

Therapy for PMS focuses on education, exercise, and diet. (Sound familiar?) It is important to realize that PMS is a common problem; it is not all in your head, and you are not just "going crazy." The education process begins with learning what is and what is not known about PMS. Current theories suggest a relationship between hormonal imbalances and PMS symptoms. However, the exact underlying abnormalities are not fully understood.

Exercise is of immediate benefit by providing an outlet for pent-up tension. Regular exercise also lessens fatigue as physical endurance increases.

The PMS prevention diet is similar to the "ideal diet" outlined in Chapter 4, "What You Should Know about the Role of Diet." This diet emphasizes whole, fresh foods, frequent small feedings, and avoiding caffeine, sugar, fat, and processed foods. I have found the craving for sweets seems to worsen the mood swings, which may be the result of erratic fluctuations in blood glucose. Eating too many sweets may also cause abdominal bloating and excessive gas, and increased salt intake invariably worsens premenstrual fluid retention. Caffeine has been implicated as a factor in breast swelling and tenderness in fibrocystic breast disease.

As part of the treatment of PMS, your physician may request that you keep a "menstrual diary" to record symptoms, daily weight, and the onset of menses. This diary may be kept in conjunction with a diet diary. The purpose of the menstrual diary is to characterize your symptoms (such as mood changes, irritability, breast swelling, and menstrual cramps) and to determine whether there is a consistent relationship between these symptoms and the menstrual cycle.

Some investigators believe that vitamin E and vitamin B_6 may help, particularly with regard to breast swelling and tenderness. Check with your physician regarding the proper dosages, since excessive amounts of vitamin B_6 may cause nerve damage. Various other vitamin and mineral supplements have been marketed in recent years for treatment of PMS. Your physician may discuss the various pharmacologic treatment modalities with you if "first-line therapy" is ineffective.

FMS

Fibromyalgia syndrome is one of the more common conditions encountered in medical practice. It belongs to the family of rheumatic diseases, which affect the joints, tendons, muscles, and ligaments. Various types of arthritis, bursitis, and tendonitis are common examples of diseases that fall into the specialty of rheumatology. Although a common cause of chronic pain and fatigue, FMS fortunately is not a degenerative, deforming process, and it is not life-threatening.

Although no direct association has been firmly established

between FMS and IBS, irritable bowel symptoms are one of the diagnostic criteria considered for the diagnosis of fibromyalgia, suggesting a possible relationship.

Dr. Don Goldenberg reported in the *Journal of the American Medical Association (JAMA)*: "Since fibromyalgia shares many common features with other poorly-described, chronic pain conditions, including. . . irritable bowel syndrome, each of these disorders should be evaluated in similar pathophysiologic fashion and compared with fibromyalgia."

Symptoms of FMS

The prominent feature of FMS is a generalized deep muscular aching discomfort in the absence of other conditions to account for these symptoms. It is similar to having a tension headache of the entire body. Although the discomfort is not always generalized, there are common so-called "trigger points" where you may note tenderness with firm pressure. These trigger points include the area between the neck and shoulders, where the knees would touch if you put them together, the back, the chest, and the buttocks. These symptoms often occur in association with headaches, disturbed sleep, morning stiffness, and fatigue.

Causes and Treatment of FMS

Although the exact cause of FMS is unknown and there is no specific test to establish the diagnosis, it may occur in association with another established rheumatic disease, such as rheumatoid arthritis. When that happens, it is referred to as secondary fibromyalgia syndrome because it occurs secondarily to an underlying condition. Symptoms of FMS may develop or worsen after an injury. In the majority of cases, symptoms simply develop and there is no associated rheumatologic disease or inciting event.

Some researchers have postulated that an underlying sleep disorder is the cause of FMS. These researchers have noted characteristic brain wave patterns in FMS patients during sleep. These patients lack Stage 4 sleep, which is the so-called "restorative phase" of sleep. Normal sleep patterns may be broadly divided into rapid eye movement (REM) and non-rapid eye movement (NREM) sleep stages. NREM sleep is divided into four successively deeper stages—Stage 4 being the deepest. FMS patients report no difficulty falling asleep, and their sleep is usually uninterrupted. They do not feel rested upon awakening, however. Normal, healthy subjects were deprived of Stage 4 sleep and developed symptoms of FMS, again suggesting a possible association.

Other possible causes of FMS include anxiety and depression, poor posture, and the normal wear and tear of aging. "Stress," which includes tension, anxiety, depression, and pent-up frustrations, will often lead to muscular aching and fatigue.

Antidepressant medications, usually in much lower doses than those employed in treating depression, are very effective for the treatment of FMS. These medications are believed to exert a beneficial effect on the disordered sleep pattern. They are most helpful if used in combination with an exercise program that increases flexibility and tone, along with some stress reduction techniques. I often use low-dose antidepressant medication as first-line pharmacologic treatment in patients with IBS who also have symptoms suggestive of FMS after they fail to improve with recommended dietary and lifestyle changes. In less severe cases, stretching exercises and relaxation therapy are all that is needed.

THE TEAM APPROACH

With multiple symptoms, you may have to decide whether a primary-care physician or a specialist is the better choice for treatment. The perspective of a primary-care physician (a general internal medicine specialist or family physician) is often different from that of a gastroenterologist. Whereas the gastroenterologist specializes in depth (within the field of gastroenterology), the primary-care physician specializes in breadth (attempting to remain current in all areas of medicine). The primary-care physician may be in a better position to recommend treatments that would, in essence, potentially correct two problems that fall within two separate specialties of medicine. For example, gastro-enterologists have special training and expertise in treating IBS, and rheumatologists have special training and expertise in treating FMS. A primary-care physician may know something about both of these disorders and thus may be the best choice for treating someone who suffers from both IBS and FMS.

With difficult cases, particularly where multiple medical problems that cross specialty designations exist, a coordinated, complementary team approach involving a primary-care physician and a specialist is often the best avenue to proper diagnosis and treatment. Many insurance companies and HMOs (health maintenance organizations) recognize this fact and now require the primary-care physician to coordinate all care given to an individual.

OTHER COEXISTING CONDITIONS

Additional disorders may occur with IBS, but it is impractical to attempt a detailed discussion of all other common medical problems that may coexist with IBS or that may be related to it in some way. There are controversial issues such as the theory of yeast overgrowth, popularized by Dr. William G. Crook in his book, *The Yeast Connection*, that could conceivably cause a variety of symptoms, including IBS. Further scientific study is needed to determine to what extent ailments may be produced by the proliferation of yeast (*Candida*) within the body. Some patients who have heard or read about the yeast-overgrowth theory have requested I prescribe anti-yeast therapy for them. I hesitate to prescribe therapy directed against a generalized overgrowth of yeast until definite benefit has been proven through well-designed studies.

Remember, a common-sense approach consisting of proper diet, exercise, and stress reduction is often all that is necessary to have a profound positive impact on both IBS and the conditions that coexist with it.

SUMMARY

Although rare, there are people who suffer combined symptoms of IBS, PMS, and FMS.

Combinations and severity of symptoms in premenstrual syndrome vary widely among women, but they generally can include mood swings, irritability and headache, menstrual cramps, bloating, fluid retention, fatigue, and craving for certain foods, often sweets.

First-line therapy for PMS focuses on education, diet, and exercise, with a prevention diet similar to the "ideal diet" outlined in Chapter 4.

Symptoms of FMS include a generalized deep muscular aching, like having a headache of the entire body. Symptoms often occur with headaches, disturbed sleep, morning stiffness, and fatigue.

Antidepressant medication has proved very effective in treating FMS.

With multiple symptoms, the combination of a primary-care physician and a specialist is often the best avenue of treatment.

A common-sense approach consisting of proper diet, exercise, and stress reduction is often all that is necessary to have a profound effect on IBS and the conditions that coexist with it.

14

OTHER COMMON GASTROINTESTINAL DISORDERS

Chapter 4, "What You Should Know about the Role of Diet," examined how the digestive system works to give you an understanding of what goes wrong when you have IBS. This chapter looks at some of the other common disorders of the gastrointestinal tract, not because you are likely to develop any of these other problems, but rather, as the saying goes, because "common things occur commonly," and these conditions may mimic or coexist with IBS.

Many of my patients, for example, have a hiatal hernia as well as IBS. Approximately 20 percent of the population has hiatal hernia. I am frequently asked questions such as: "The upper GI showed a hiatal hernia—is this the cause of my problem?" and "How is IBS different?"

Hemorrhoids are another very common problem that in my experience does seem to be more prevalent in IBS patients. The reason may be that diarrhea and constipation aggravate "piles." Since I frequently counsel patients on how to deal with this "pain in the butt," a word about hemorrhoids is appropriate in a book on IBS.

On a positive note, IBS does not predispose you to colon cancer or colitis. These conditions are mentioned simply for general interest and knowledge.

It is important for everyone to be aware of colon cancer, since it is the second most frequent cause of death from cancer in North America, after lung cancer. Should your IBS symptoms change and you develop symptoms such as weight loss, bleeding from the rectum, or change in bowel habits or stool caliber, see your doctor immediately! Do not assume it is "simply my IBS." Although you are no more likely to develop colon cancer or polyps than anyone else, the fact that you have IBS does not protect you from colon cancer or any other common gastrointestinal malady.

Our review begins at the upper end of the gastrointestinal tract and works down to the rectum. Then the gallbladder is reviewed, and finally infections of the gastrointestinal tract are discussed. Remember, this chapter is not an all-inclusive review of every condition that affects the gastrointestinal system but is intended to take some of the mystery out of the common medical problems that affect your gut.

REFLUX ESOPHAGITIS

Did you know that heartburn has nothing to do with your heart? Terms such as "heartburn" and "indigestion" mean different things to different people. For some, "heartburn" refers to that uncomfortable feeling you may experience when you eat too much or too fast. For others, heartburn is an intense burning pain in the upper abdomen and mid-chest that may be associated with a sour taste in the mouth. Physicians technically refer to this condition as reflux esophagitis.

Causes and Diagnosis of Reflux Esophagitis

As the name implies, the acid contents of the stomach flow back into the esophagus, leading, over time, to inflammation of the esophagus, which in turn leads to esophagitis. Eating too much or too fast may predispose some people to an occasional bout of "acid indigestion." For others, this is a chronic and recurring problem.

A circular ring of muscle divides the lower esophagus from the stomach. This ring, referred to as the lower esophageal sphincter (LES), normally remains contracted and prevents the acid contents of the stomach from moving upward into the esophagus. The swallowing mechanism allows for relaxation of the LES during swallowing. However, if the LES relaxes at other times, regurgitation may occur and heartburn results.

The diagnosis of reflux esophagitis is suggested by the symptoms. X rays of the upper gastrointestinal tract or direct observation through endoscopy help confirm the diagnosis.

Treatment of Reflux Esophagitis

Several general recommendations are often helpful in reducing the frequency and severity of reflux esophagitis symptoms. For obese patients, losing weight tends to reduce abdominal pressure. At the same time, these patients should avoid tight-fitting garments or any activities that increase abdominal pressure. Elevating the head of the bed six to eight inches by placing blocks under the bedpost or frame allows gravity to work for you at night. Sufferers should also avoid stooping or bending shortly after a meal, since these movements encourage reflux into the esophagus.

Foods to avoid include fatty foods, chocolates, alcohol, citrus fruit juices, and coffee. Nicotine in any form, but especially cigarettes, decreases LES tone and should be avoided. Avoid late-night snacks, heavy meals, or lying down shortly after meals. Antacids, which neutralize acid in the esophagus and stomach, are helpful. Take these on an as-needed basis; they usually provide immediate relief. Your doctor may also prescribe medications designed to block acid secretion in the stomach. In rare instances, surgery may be required to treat resistant cases.

If the problem is allowed to continue untreated, the esophagus may eventually scar and develop a stricture. Repeated acid irritation of the esophagus may also predispose the sufferer to cancer of the esophagus. This very serious disorder led to John Wayne's death. If you experience difficulty in swallowing or the sensation that food is getting stuck as it goes down, see your physician immediately; these symptoms may indicate stricture formation or esophageal cancer.

Coexistence with Hiatal Hernia

Reflux esophagitis may be associated with a hiatal hernia, the protrusion of a portion of the stomach through the diaphragm into the chest. I have heard patients refer to this common problem as their "high hernia." Hiatal hernias become more common with aging and can occur in up to 70 percent of those over age 60. Most hiatal hernias produce no symptoms, and no treatment is required.

If a patient with reflux has a hiatal hernia, the treatment is the same as for a patient with reflux who does not have a hiatal hernia. Patients with hiatal hernias seem to complain more of bloating after meals and are more likely to experience the relatively uncommon problem of esophageal spasm. When asked what it felt like, one of my patients with this disorder explained: "It is like a charley horse in the center of my chest."

PEPTIC ULCER DISEASE

Unlike the esophagus, which is damaged by acid, the stomach is designed to tolerate, under normal circumstances, the acid produced by specialized cells within the stomach. Peptic ulcers are raw areas that develop either in the stomach (gastric ulcers) or the first part of the small intestine (duodenal ulcers). These raw areas are similar to the mouth ulcers or "canker sores" that many people experience at some time.

Symptoms and Causes of Peptic Ulcers

As the stomach acid infiltrates the raw area, an intense, burning pain may be felt, usually just below the breastbone. It is like pouring salt on an open wound. Most, but not all, ulcers produce symptoms that are variously described as "gnawing pains" and "hunger pains." The term "hunger pain" probably arises from the observation that eating food or drinking milk will often temporarily relieve symptoms. The food or milk simply coats the stomach and neutralizes the acid.

Ulcer pain frequently occurs at night when the stomach is empty. This is in contrast to the pain of IBS, which experts contend should rarely, if ever, awaken a patient from sleep.

What causes peptic ulcers? The answer to this question has been debated for some time. The current thinking is that under ordinary circumstances there is a balance between appropriate acid production and the stomach lining's defensive mucosal protection against self-digestion by the acid produced. The scale could be tipped in either direction by an excess of acid production or a breakdown in the mucosal barrier.

Emotional stress and smoking may lead to excessive acid production and result in peptic ulcers. Breakdown in the mucosal barriers may occur as a result of taking an anti-inflammatory medication used to treat arthritis and pain. Examples include over-the-counter products, in addition to many prescription medications collectively referred to as NSAIDs (Non-Steroidal Anti-Inflammatory Drugs). Fortunately, there is a new medication to help prevent ulcer formation in those patients predisposed to ulcers who, at the same time, require arthritis medications.

Another recent breakthrough in the study of ulcer disease is the discovery of an organism called *Helicobacter pyloris* (previously referred to as *Campylobacter pyloris*), which has been identified as a possible cause of mucosal damage, gastritis, and peptic ulceration. In fact, some resistant peptic ulcers have been successfully treated with antibiotics aimed at eradicating this organism.

Treatment of Peptic Ulcers

Bland diets are no longer recommended for patients with ulcer disease. I tell my patients to avoid only those foods that seem to aggravate symptoms. With many patients, the avoidance of very hot or very spicy foods is all that is necessary as an "ulcer diet."

Most physicians continue to treat peptic ulcers with conventional therapy consisting of antacids to neutralize stomach acid, medications designed to decrease acid production, or medications that assist the mucosal defense barriers.

Similar Conditions

Some patients have burning pains, belching, and bloating suggestive of peptic ulcers, but no ulcer is evident by X ray or endoscopy. Physicians believe that these patients have so-called "nonulcer dyspepsia." These patients may have low-grade inflammation of the stomach or duodenum, which responds to acid-blocking medication. Alternatively, they may have a disorder of stomach motility that is responsive to promotility medications.

INTESTINAL ADHESIONS

As partially digested food, referred to as chyme, exits the stomach, it enters the small intestine. The small intestine is where the problem of adhesions usually occurs. Adhesions are abnormal fibrous bands or scars that develop between internal organs. Often these bands form between contiguous loops of small intestine, causing these same loops to stick together. If you were to observe a surgeon perform a laparotomy (surgery of the abdominal cavity) under ordinary circumstances, you would note the surgeon freely move around or shift the 21 feet of small intestine. Were that same surgeon operating on a patient with adhesions, you would notice that certain portions of the intestine adhere to one another. The significance of adhesions is that they may interfere with the normal peristaltic activity of the small intestine, the rhythmic contractions that move the chyme through the intestine. Interruption of these contractions can lead to intermittent abdominal pain. In some cases, the intestine can become kinked, resulting in an intestinal obstruction.

Causes and Diagnosis of Intestinal Adhesions

Adhesions most commonly occur some time after a surgical operation. Just as visible scars form on the abdomen during the healing process, scars may form internally as healing progresses. Infections or inflammation of the abdominal cavity increase the likelihood that adhesions will form. For example, surgery for a ruptured appendix, wherein infected material has infiltrated the abdominal cavity, is much more likely to produce adhesions than an appendectomy performed before rupture occurs.

Unfortunately, there is no simple way to determine if adhesions are present without direct visual observation through a laparoscope or during exploratory surgery. And the presence of adhesions is not proof positive they are causing the problem. An upper GI series with small-bowel follow-through may occasionally be helpful in making this determination. I have seen IBS symptoms worsen in numerous patients after an abdominal operation for an unrelated condition. I theorize that in these patients fibrous adhesions of the small intestine may be a cofactor that further interferes with intestinal motility and contributes to worsening symptoms.

Treatment of Intestinal Adhesions

Exploratory or laparoscopic surgery is the only effective treatment for adhesions. Cutting through the adhesive bands may eliminate the problem. Unfortunately, since surgery causes adhesions, there is always risk of recurrence later.

SPIGELIAN HERNIA

Spigelian hernias are not really a gastrointestinal disorder but occur as a result of a protrusion of the intestinal contents through a weak area in the lower lateral abdominal wall. I have found this condition to be more common than the medical literature suggests. At the same time, it is difficult to diagnose; one surgeon reported he was able to secure diagnosis before surgery in only 50 percent of his cases.

The key to diagnosis is recurrent pain and tenderness localized within the abdominal wall. A bulge may be noted, particularly when standing and straining. Symptoms may simulate an intra-abdominal condition, and I have seen patients unfortunately misdiagnosed as having IBS since no other cause for their recurrent pain could be identified.

One factor that predisposes one to the development of spigelian hernia is an abdominal incision, particularly a transverse lower abdominal incision made at the time of a caesarean delivery. Treatment for spigelian hernia is surgical repair.

DIVERTICULOSIS/DIVERTICULITIS

Undigested material from the small intestine is propelled forward into the colon or large intestine. It is in the colon where diverticulosis, or the appearance of small outpouchings called diverticula, occurs. The condition becomes more common as people age. Whereas half the population over age 60 has diverticula, they are rare in those under age 30.

Causes of Diverticula

Diverticula are thought to form over time as the result of weakening in the colon wall where blood vessels exist, much as a weak spot might occur in the wall of an inner tube or tire. Diverticulosis is common in industrialized nations such as the United States and Canada and correspondingly rare in Asia, Africa, and other developing areas. Authorities theorize that a relative lack of dietary fiber in industrialized nations contributes to the development of diverticulosis, which is unseen in countries where whole grains are the largest constituent of diet. The theory is that adding bulk to the stool actually decreases intracolonic pressure, making weak spots and "blowouts" less likely.

Symptoms of Diverticulosis

When diverticula occur in the absence of inflammation, the condition is referred to as diverticulosis. Diverticulosis often produces no symptoms. When symptoms do occur, the usual manifestations are episodic, crampy lower abdominal pain, gas, bloating, and irregular bowel movements: symptoms that mimic IBS. Additionally, diverticulosis may occasionally cause rectal bleeding. See your doctor immediately if this occurs.

Symptoms of Diverticulitis

If a diverticulum ruptures, then intracolonic bacteria are released into the normal sterile abdominal cavity, causing infection and inflammation—referred to as diverticulitis. The symptoms of diverticulitis include fever, abdominal pain, and abdominal tenderness. The pain and tenderness are usually felt in the left lower abdomen, since diverticula are more common in that area of the colon on the left, referred to as the sigmoid colon. Fortunately, diverticulitis is a relatively rare complication of diverticulosis, occurring in fewer than 15 percent of all persons with diverticula.

Diagnosis and Treatment

The presence of diverticula is easily detected by barium-enema X rays or direct observation during endoscopy (sigmoidoscopy or colonoscopy). Treatment for diverticulosis consists of a gradual increase in dietary fiber to decrease intracolonic pressure. Antispasmodics may be used symptomatically to treat the associated cramps. For diverticulitis, antibiotics are prescribed to treat the infection. If oral antibiotics are inadequate, hospitalization, intravenous antibiotics, and occasionally surgery may be required.

INFLAMMATORY BOWEL DISEASE (IBD)

Ulcerative colitis and Crohn's disease are chronic inflammatory intestinal conditions of unknown cause. These two disorders are often collectively referred to as inflammatory bowel disease, or IBD. The major difference between the two disorders is that ulcerative colitis is limited to the colon and rectum, whereas Crohn's disease (also referred to as regional enteritis) may affect any segment of the alimentary canal, from the esophagus to the anus. Crohn's disease commonly affects the last portion of the small intestine, referred to as the ileum.

Symptoms of the two disorders are variable, depending on the severity of the disease and which areas are affected. Mild cases are associated with diarrhea and crampy abdominal pain. Bloody diarrhea, fever, and weight loss are seen with more serious cases. Unlike IBS, which does not predispose one to cancer, ulcerative colitis is associated with an increased risk of colon cancer.

The diagnosis of IBD is supported by characteristic X-ray findings and is usually confirmed by the pathologist's review of biopsy specimens obtained during endoscopy. Orally and rectally administered corticosteriods are generally prescribed for treatment. Surgery may be necessary in severe cases, particularly with ulcerative colitis.

COLON CANCER/POLYPS

Some experts contend that in addition to ulcerative colitis, a lack of dietary fiber also predisposes one to the development of colon cancer. Certain types of colon polyps (small, fleshy, mushroom-shaped growths), if left alone, will undergo malignant, cancerous transformation. Colon cancer is very common, with more than 120,000 new cases diagnosed in North America each year. With early detection, the potential for saving lives from this disease is great. The methods of early detection consist of digital rectum exam (in which the physician inserts a gloved index finger into the rectum), testing for occult blood in the stool, and screening sigmoidoscopy. Some of the presenting symptoms of colon cancer may consist of change in bowel habits, abdominal discomfort, rectal bleeding, weakness secondary to anemia, and weight loss.

The diagnosis is made by X rays or endoscopy of the colon. If premalignant polyps are found, they are usually removed through the colonoscope by a procedure referred to as polypectomy. Follow-up surveillance exams are recommended to detect any recurrences. Colon cancer is usually treated with surgery, sometimes combined with chemotherapy or radiation therapy.

APPENDICITIS

While evaluating patients with abdominal pain, I am frequently asked: "Could this be my appendix?" Certainly, this is one of the more common causes of belly pain. Just about everyone knows someone who has had his or her appendix removed. After all, this four-inch dead-end pouch attached to the cecum (the first part of the colon) serves no known useful purpose and frequently becomes infected, causing appendicitis.

Problems of the appendix are not usually chronic and recurring. Rather, acute appendicitis will occur for no particular reason, causing pain that initially is around the umbilicus (belly button) and, as it becomes more intense, will localize to the right lower abdomen. The pain is usually accompanied by fever and a very tender tummy. No special tests are required to make the diagnosis, although an elevated white blood cell count is certainly supportive evidence. When appendicitis is suspected in a relatively sick individual, immediate surgery is usually recommended to remove the appendix before it ruptures.

HEMORRHOIDS

Hemorrhoids (piles) are one of the more common problems of the digestive tract. Because diarrhea and constipation aggravate the problem, the discomfort of hemorrhoids is especially common in patients with IBS. In addition to causing rectal pain and bleeding, hemorrhoids are a source of embarrassment to many.

I recall one patient who developed a severe case of hemorrhoids while on his honeymoon. It seems he was prone to constipation while traveling, and the constipation, with its resultant straining during bowel movements, resulted in "piles of piles." Well, so much for the horseback riding excursions on that trip...

Frequently patients come in petrified with fear because they have experienced their first bout of rectal bleeding, which turned out to be secondary to hemorrhoids. Although hemorrhoids are a common cause of rectal bleeding, do not assume that they are always the cause. Consult your physician to make certain, as rectal cancer and polyps may also cause bleeding from the rectum. Your doctor may perform an anuscopy or sigmoidoscopy to make this determination.

Symptoms of Hemorrhoids

What, exactly, are hemorrhoids? Simply stated, hemorrhoids are dilated veins around the rectum and anus. When they occur outside the anus they are referred to as external hemorrhoids.

133

The skin overlying external hemorrhoids is very sensitive; therefore, the most common manifestation is pain. A tender lump may be felt when you are bathing.

Internal hemorrhoids occur inside the rectum and do not generally produce pain unless they "pooch out" or prolapse. When internal hemorrhoids prolapse outside the rectum, the anus may close, causing strangulation or thrombosis of the blood vessel. This can be very painful.

Internal hemorrhoids are more likely to bleed, and this may be the only clue to their presence. In addition to pain and bleeding, hemorrhoids may also cause rectal itching when they become irritated, and soiling of the undergarments with mucus or feces, since the swollen veins may prevent complete closure of the anus. Hemorrhoids may be associated with painful anal fissures, which are cracks in the sensitive skin around the anus. Skin tags may form around the anus if the skin overlying the hemorrhoids becomes stretched.

Causes of Hemorrhoids

You may be wondering by now what causes hemorrhoids. This is an area of much debate. Conditions that cause increased pressure on the veins in the abdomen, such as pregnancy, are thought to contribute. Varicose veins of the legs are more common with subsequent pregnancies, and hemorrhoids may be likened to varicose veins of the rectum. You can thank your parents for this, since there does seem to be a genetic predisposition to this condition. Straining to pass a large, hard stool, or frequent diarrheal stools, may, as a result of pressure and shearing forces, aggravate the condition. I do not think hemorrhoids are an occupational hazard for truck drivers, but certainly jobs that require prolonged periods of sitting may compound the discomfort.

Treatment of Hemorrhoids

Fortunately, hemorrhoids usually respond to conservative treatment. I recommend the following:

- Avoid constipation or diarrhea. This may be accomplished by increasing dietary fiber. Use of a "bulking agent" such as natural psyllium may be helpful in normalizing stools by virtue of its water-retaining properties. Products such as these will soften a hard stool and firm up a loose stool.
- Avoid straining during bowel movements. When hemorrhoids are present, you may experience a fullness or what is referred to as a sense of incomplete evacuation after a bowel movement. You may push and strain to get this last bit of stool out when, in fact, all of the stool is gone and further straining will only push the hemorrhoids out, causing prolapse.
- Take a sitz bath. Fill the bathtub with just enough very warm water to cover the rectal area. Sit in the tub for a few minutes until the water cools. Do this as often as your schedule permits. Ideally, a sitz bath after each bowel movement would provide optimal cleaning and soothing of the rectal area. If you are plagued with hemorrhoids, consider installing a bidet.
- If you are unable to take a sitz bath or cannot afford to install a bidet, try cleansing with one of the various medicated pads or cotton soaked in witch hazel to help ease discomfort.

In addition to the above "home remedies," your doctor may prescribe some hydrocortisone-containing preparations. When all else fails, a referral to a surgeon may be indicated for one of the various therapeutic techniques that provide more definitive treatment. Severe pain may develop if a blood clot or thrombosis develops in a hemorrhoid. This occurrence frequently requires surgical intervention.

PROCTALGIA FUGAX

Some people believe that the sudden onset of intense rectal pain—referred to as *proctalgia fugax*—is in some way related to

IBS. There does seem to be a higher incidence of this complaint among IBS sufferers. The pain is usually described as a spasm or a cramp. Although the cause is unknown, symptoms are thought to result from spasm of the muscles around the anus, like a charley horse. A hot sitz bath may relieve the discomfort. Occasionally, medications may be prescribed if symptoms are severe or frequent.

GALLSTONES

Gallstones are a relatively common cause of abdominal distress. These stones form in a saclike structure called the gallbladder, which is located under the liver. The gallbladder stores the bile manufactured by the liver until it is needed in the small intestine to aid in fat digestion. When called on, the gallbladder contracts to squirt bile into the intestine. If the gallbladder contains stones, the stones may block the flow of bile, resulting in a rather intense pain in the mid-upper or upper right abdomen.

Pain is classically worse after a meal that is high in fat. In less severe cases, nonspecific symptoms such as belching, bloating, and gas may occur: symptoms that commonly occur in IBS patients. The majority of patients with gallstones are asymptomatic, which is to say their gallstones produce no symptoms.

Cholesterol is a major constituent of bile, and most gallstones form because the concentration of cholesterol in the bile is too high. Heredity, advancing age, being a female, and pregnancy are all risk factors for the development of gallstones.

The traditional treatment for symptomatic gallstones has been surgical removal, or cholecystectomy. Recent advances in the treatment of gallstone disease include mechanical breakdown of stones using sound waves during a procedure referred to as lithotripsy. Drugs that slowly dissolve stones, and newer surgical techniques such as laparoscopic laser cholecystectomy, are also used. Each of these newer techniques has certain limitations that require individualized recommendations for specific treatment by your physician. If cholecystitis (infection of the gallbladder) develops, then emergency cholecystectomy, using customary techniques, is usually required.

GIARDIASIS

Infections of the gastrointestinal tract may produce symptoms such as cramps, diarrhea, bloating, and gas. One such infection is due to a common intestinal parasite called *Giardia*. Giardiasis is being recognized more frequently as a cause of acute and chronic diarrheal illness with higher than average prevalence in the Rocky Mountain region where I practice. The illness may begin suddenly or gradually and may last for days, weeks, or if it becomes chronic, years. Symptoms may occur daily or only intermittently.

As part of an evaluation of IBS, your doctor may ask you to submit one or several stool specimens so that he or she may look for *Giardia* and other possible causes of gastrointestinal infections. A difficulty arises from the fact that the *Giardia* cyst may be easily missed by standard stool examinations. The chance of spotting the cyst is increased by evaluating more than one specimen, but even after three separate specimens are checked, there is approximately a 15 percent chance that diagnosis will be missed in patients with established giardiasis. Fortunately, there is a newer method of stool analysis, which is purported to detect the *Giardia* antigen in most cases with a single stool sample.

As of this writing, there is no definite test to absolutely exclude the possibility of *Giardia*. If giardiasis is suspected, your doctor may elect to prescribe an antibiotic and treat you empirically, without establishing a firm diagnosis. This decision may spare you the trouble of having to play amateur scatologist and study your excrement. It may turn out that as our present knowledge of IBS increases, researchers will discover other intestinal infections that may be the real cause of symptoms in patients previously labeled as having IBS.

SUMMARY

Other common gastrointestinal disorders that may mimic or co-exist with IBS include appendicitis, colon cancer, intestinal adhesions, diverticulosis, gallstones, giardiasis, hiatal hernia, inflammatory bowel disease, intestinal adhesions, peptic ulcer disease, polyps, *proctalgia fugax*, and reflux esophagitis.

15

COMMON TESTS
YOU MAY FACE

This chapter discusses common tests used to evaluate the gastrointestinal system and to diagnose disorders that may mimic IBS. (Please refer to Chapter 14, "Other Common Gastrointestinal Disorders," for a discussion of other common gastrointestinal disorders your doctor may be attempting to rule out.) The chapter does not contain an exhaustive listing of every test used to evaluate the gastrointestinal system, only the more common ones. The intent is to provide some insight into how the various tests are performed and what kind of information is obtained by performing the tests.

Knowing what to expect will help allay your fears if you must undergo any of these evaluations. Your physician will determine which test to order, if any. Understand that you will probably not have occasion to take all the tests mentioned. At the same time, some tests may be ordered that are not covered here. The chapter first looks at radiographic or X-ray tests of the gastrointestinal tract, then reviews endoscopic procedures, and concludes with miscellaneous tests.

RADIOGRAPHIC (OR IMAGING) TECHNIQUES

Most of the following tests are performed in a hospital radiology department. The tests are taken and interpreted by a radiologist, a medical doctor with specialized training and expertise in X-ray procedures. Upon completion of the tests, the radiologist sends a complete report to your physician.

The specialty of radiology is relatively new; the specialty board, which certifies doctors as specialists in the field of radiology, was founded in 1934. Since that time, great advances have been made, such as the development of the CAT (Computerized Axial Tomography) scan and MRI (Magnetic Resonance Imagery) scanners.

These specialized "cameras" produce detailed pictures of internal structures. However, most X-ray procedures of the gastrointestinal (GI) tract utilize more conventional X-ray machines. With these machines, contrast material (usually barium) is either swallowed (as for an upper GI series) or inserted into the rectum through a small tube (for a barium-enema or lower GI series) to increase opacity and contrast on the X-ray film.

Upper GI Series

An upper GI is an X-ray study used to evaluate the first part of the digestive tract, which includes the esophagus, stomach, and duodenum. In this test, you are asked to swallow barium (a chalky liquid) and possibly to ingest some powder that produces air in the stomach. The barium coats the inside of the intestine, outlining its contours and any irregularities of this hollow structure. As you swallow the liquid, the radiologist watches on a fluoroscope, which is an X-ray television apparatus. You are asked to turn from side to side as the X-ray technologist takes several "still" pictures of your stomach. After the films are processed, the radiologist reviews them for the presence of swallowing disorders, ulcers, inflammation, hiatal hernia, and tumors.

You may not eat or drink for eight hours before the test, since the presence of any food in the stomach will interfere with the image. For the most part, the test is not too trying and is over in 30 to 45 minutes or less. Granted, barium is not very tasty and the exam table is rather hard. Sometimes the upper GI is followed by a further examination of your small intestine called a small-bowel series or small-bowel follow-through. This test usually follows an upper GI, but it may be ordered as a separate examination if the doctor suspects an abnormality of the small intestine (such as Crohn's disease or adhesions). If the test is to view the entire small bowel, then X-rays will be taken every 15 to 30 minutes as the barium moves from the stomach through your intestines, in the same way food moves through the system during digestion.

The examination may take from 30 minutes to several hours, depending on the transit time of your digestive tract. The average is 1 1/2 to 2 hours. You will wait in the radiology department between films, so take plenty of reading material or handwork to pass the time if your doctor orders a small-bowel series. Preparation for a small-bowel series is the same as that for an upper GI series, requiring that you fast for 8 hours before the test.

Barium-Enema or Lower GI Series

The barium-enema or lower GI series is an X-ray examination of the colon or large intestine. It may detect disorders of the colon such as cancer, polyps, diverticulitis, inflammatory bowel disease, and obstruction. Since the large intestine must be free of fecal material before the exam, you will be asked to follow a limited diet (usually liquids only) and take laxative preparations the day before. You are probably thinking, "Limited diet, laxative preparations—I do not like this test and I have not had it yet."

Well, if you survive the prep, which is not exactly as bad as it sounds, you will likely find the exam undignified and somewhat unpleasant, but not particularly painful. A plain X-ray film of the abdomen is taken before the exam. During the exam, you lie on your side and the doctor inserts a small, lubricated plastic tube into your rectum. Barium is introduced into the tube and slowly fills your colon. The flow of barium is monitored on a fluoroscope. Often air is pumped into the colon to produce an air-contrast or double-contrast study. You will be asked to turn from side to side and roll from your back to your stomach as the air-barium mixture coats the lining of your colon. Multiple X-ray pictures will be taken.

As the barium enters the colon, you may feel the urge for a bowel movement. A small balloon around the plastic tube helps prevent the barium from backing out, but do not be embarrassed if some of the barium does leak out; technologists and radiologists are accustomed to this. You may also experience some cramping and bloating as the procedure progresses. Afterwards, you will be invited to visit the rest room to evacuate the barium and air. ("Oh what a relief. . . ") A final, "empty" X-ray will be taken.

The entire test usually takes 20 to 30 minutes. Your stools may remain white and chalky for one or two days following the exam as you expel the remainder of the barium. Maintain an adequate fluid intake afterwards because barium can cause constipation.

ABDOMINAL ULTRASOUND (SONOGRAM)

Ultrasound utilizes sound waves to produce images of structures within the abdomen. It is a safe, painless, effective way to evaluate intra-abdominal organs such as the gallbladder, liver, and pancreas. In many cases it is replacing the oral cholecystogram and becoming the procedure of choice for detecting gallstones.

Unlike the oral cholecystogram, the ultrasound exam does not expose you to radiation. In addition, no dye is used, so you don't have to worry about allergic reactions to iodine. The downside is that the high-frequency sound waves emitted from the transducer do not penetrate air spaces well, so the exam is of no value in detecting abnormalities of the intestine. I know—you were thinking, "Great! I will just have an ultrasound rather than a barium enema." Sorry. If an abnormality of the intestinal tract is suspected, you may well need the GI series. The ultrasound exam is also technically difficult to perform on obese patients or on patients with scars or bandages on the abdomen.

For a gallbladder ultrasound, you must refrain from eating or drinking for eight hours beforehand. Ideally, the gallbladder will be distended with bile. Since the gallbladder contracts after a meal, you are asked to fast before this procedure.

Before the exam, the technologist places a jellylike material on your abdomen to improve contact with the transducer, which is the scanner that will be moved across your abdomen. Images appear on a television screen as the sound waves painlessly penetrate certain tissue and then bounce back to the transducer. Several still pictures are taken as part of the permanent record and for later review by a radiologist. If it sounds simple, that is because it really is.

ENDOSCOPY

Endoscopy is a procedure that allows the physician to directly view the upper or lower digestive tract. The instrument used is a flexible, fiberoptic tube that has a light source and various channels through which air or water may be introduced or removed and through which biopsy specimens may be taken. The type of exam and scope are determined by which portion of the alimentary canal is to be examined. For example, with sigmoidoscopy, doctors use a sigmoidoscope to observe the rectum and lower portion of the large intestine (sigmoid colon). If it is necessary to observe the entire large intestine, a longer scope (approximately six feet), referred to as a colonoscope, is used. For evaluation of the upper digestive tract, an esophagogastroduodenoscopy (EGD) is performed to evaluate the esophagus, stomach, and duodenum. Although the technology is available to directly view the approximately 21 feet of small intestine, small-bowel endoscopy (enteroscopy) is impractical and only experimental at this point.

Your doctor may suggest endoscopy to more closely examine abnormalities noted on X-ray examinations or to detect minor abnormalities such as inflammation, which may not be seen with X-ray. Endoscopy also allows an opportunity for collecting biopsy specimens for pathologic evaluation. Through the endoscope, small polyps may be removed from the colon, and foreign objects that have lodged in the esophagus may be removed.

Rare complications of endoscopy include bleeding and perforation of the intestine (which may require emergency surgery). The procedure is usually performed in the endoscopy lab (also known as the butts and guts room) of a hospital or outpatient clinic.

Esophagogastroduodenoscopy (EGD)

This procedure may be recommended to look for the presence of swallowing disorders, hiatal hernia, ulcers, tumors, and bleeding or inflammation of the esophagus, stomach, or duodenum. The procedure is usually performed by a gastroenterologist, a medical doctor with special training in the treatment of gastrointestinal disorders. You will be asked not to eat or drink for several hours before the test so that the stomach will be empty. Your throat will be sprayed with a topical anesthetic to numb it and decrease the gag reflex. Although you will not be "put to sleep," some IV sedation is usually given to make you groggy. The procedure is not painful, and patients always have the option to use only the spray. Some technologists report that adequate instruction and explanation are often adequate anesthesia. Under sedation, however, you may not remember much that happens after this point.

A mouthpiece is placed between the teeth, and the scope gradually advances through the back of the throat and into the esophagus. The physician will view, in turn, the esophagus, stomach, and duodenum through an eyepiece or on a video monitor. Any suspicious areas may be biopsied. If the physician notes a bleeding site, it may be cauterized through the scope. An entire routine procedure lasts 15 to 30 minutes. It will take longer for the sedation to wear off, so you must have someone assist you home.

Flexible Sigmoidoscopy

Flexible sigmoidoscopy is used to evaluate the rectum and lower colon. Many primary-care physicians, such as family physicians and internists, are trained in this procedure; it is technically less difficult than an EGD or a colonoscopy. The procedure is frequently recommended for screening for colorectal cancer and polyps. It can also detect abnormalities such as hemorrhoids, inflammation, and diverticula. The procedure is generally carried out in the doctor's office. One or more enemas just before the procedure is usually all the preparation necessary. Sedation, with its potential complications, is usually not required with sigmoidoscopy, since it is generally well tolerated. (I did not say you would enjoy it.)

The test begins when you are asked to lie on your left side with your knees pulled up toward your chest. The doctor inspects the exterior of the anus and performs a manual exam of the rectum before inserting the scope. After lubricating the tip of the scope, the doctor will gently ease it into the rectum. Air is introduced to expand the bowel and make viewing easier. The air may occasionally cause a crampy discomfort, and you may experience a strong urge to defecate. Do not become embarrassed if some of the air escapes; it is odorless. Although most patients easily endure the procedure, should it become intolerable, let your physician know. Air can be suctioned out of the bowel and the procedure briefly interrupted. In most cases, the crampy discomfort will ease and the procedure can continue from that point. If you are experiencing discomfort, it often helps to take slow, deep breaths and try to relax. The procedure usually lasts 15 to 30 minutes.

If your physician notes any polyps or suspicious areas, biopsies may be taken. Biopsies are painless.

Colonoscopy

The longer colonoscope allows direct viewing of the entire colon. Colonoscopy, usually performed by a gastroenterologist, detects the same disorders noted with flexible sigmoidoscopy. The difference is that more of the colon can be viewed with colonoscopy.

Since more of the colon is involved, preparation for colonoscopy is more complex. You are given a bowel-cleansing preparation the afternoon before the test and are restricted to liquids after completing the prep. IV sedation may be offered, since colonoscopy causes more discomfort than sigmoidoscopy. The basic technique and procedure for colonoscopy is similar to that of flexible sigmoidoscopy. The entire procedure usually takes approximately one hour.

MISCELLANEOUS TESTS

Hydrogen Breath Test

One other test has proved useful to me in evaluating patients with suspected lactose intolerance or sensitivity. Ordinarily, a lactose-restricted diet (see pages 182-83) for two to three weeks is all that is necessary to determine the presence of lactose intolerance or sensitivity. (If an intolerance exists, lactase enzyme supplements should help correct the problem.) I have encountered many patients for whom the evidence presents a confusing picture. One such patient determined that he was intolerant of dairy products and had, for some time, avoided all milk, cheese, ice cream, and so on. I suggested he try lactase enzyme supplements. He did, and found them ineffective. At this point, I began to suspect he might not be lactose intolerant, so I suggested we perform a hydrogen breath test.

The hydrogen breath test is an accurate, simple test for evaluating lactose intolerance. The patient ingests a test dose of lactose. At periodic intervals—usually 30 minutes—the patient is asked to breathe into a unit where a sample of the breath is collected and analyzed for hydrogen content.

In lactose-intolerant individuals, lactose is not broken down and absorbed in the small intestine. Unabsorbed lactose is eventually broken down by bacteria in the colon, producing hydrogen gas. Some of this gas enters the bloodstream and can be detected as an elevated hydrogen content in expired breath. Normal individuals exhibit only a trace of hydrogen after a lactose load. The test is usually performed in a hospital GI lab or outpatient clinic and lasts two to four hours. Fructose and sorbitol malabsorption are also determined by use of breath hydrogen analysis.

As for the patient mentioned earlier, the hydrogen breath test was normal, indicating no lactose intolerance. Further dairy product challenges revealed that he only had a problem with cheese, ice cream, and whole milk. He could tolerate skim milk well; I suspect it was the high fat content of cheese, ice cream, and whole milk that caused his symptoms and not the lactose content. He has begun to enjoy skim milk with his morning cereal and tolerates low-fat cheeses quite well.

Blood Tests

The erythrocyte sedimentation rate (ESR) is a blood test that indicates whether or not inflammation is present in the body. The ESR does not identify the source of the inflammation but may be a clue to the presence of inflammatory bowel disease. Routine blood tests may reveal presence of kidney disease, liver disease, or electrolyte abnormalities.

Examination of Stool Samples

Stool sample examination—preferably a watery one—helps in detecting such problems as infection of the bowel. The stool is analyzed for presence of blood, white blood cells (pus cells), ova, and parasites. The sample is cultured to detect disease-causing organisms such as *Salmonella*. Excessive amounts of fat in the stool may indicate problems with malabsorption, such as those seen with disease of the pancreas.

Remember, in most cases the history (a detailed account of your symptoms) will provide the best clues as to the cause of your problem. Various tests may be used to refute or confirm suspicions or to rule out certain disorders with symptoms overlapping those of IBS. It is usually not necessary to perform every test possible to rule out every possible disorder that may simulate IBS. It is unfortunate that there is not a single test to "rule in" and definitely identify the presence of IBS. Until there is, be patient when working with your doctor in an attempt to "get to the bottom of it."

SUMMARY

A battery of tests is utilized to identify other disorders that may cause some of the symptoms of IBS.

Radiographic or imaging techniques produce X rays of the intestinal tract. The upper GI series uses X rays to evaluate the first part of the digestive tract, and the lower GI series uses X rays to examine the colon or large intestine.

Abdominal ultrasound uses sound waves to examine the abdomen and evaluate the gallbladder, liver, and pancreas.

In endoscopy, physicians use a tube or scope to directly view the upper and lower digestive tract. In an EGD (esophagogastroduodenoscopy), a tube is inserted down the throat and into the esophagus so that the physician can observe the esophagus, stomach, and duodenum. Flexible sigmoidoscopy uses a tube inserted into the rectum to evaluate the rectum and lower colon. Colonoscopy allows direct viewing of the entire colon through a tube inserted into the rectum.

Miscellaneous tests such as the hydrogen breath test, special blood tests, and stool samples can be used to evaluate the gastrointestinal system.

CONCLUSION

IBS can affect every aspect of your life, including your daily routines, your personal outlook, and your enjoyment of sex. Although the exact causes of IBS remain unknown and treatment is symptomatic, the key to obtaining relief is to assess your situation, then take calculated steps to minimize the more troublesome symptoms. The most important component of a healthful lifestyle is the conviction that improvement is possible. Be patient with yourself; it is difficult to change habits overnight. Some key considerations for IBS sufferers include:

- Make necessary changes in your diet and lifestyle to minimize annoying symptoms and improve total health.
- Avoid the three social drugs: alcohol, nicotine, and caffeine.
- Learn to practice stress reduction techniques to give your body a chance to cope with daily pressures.
- Increase your level of physical activity.

We invite your comments and questions. Please make a copy of and fill out the reader comment page at the end of this book, and send it to us (or any other questions or comments you may have).

APPENDIX 1

QUESTIONNAIRES

1. How long have you had abdominal pain?
2. Do you have more than one pain? Yes ☐   No ☐
   If so, how many different pains do you have?
3. Where is the worst pain located?
4. How often does the pain occur, and how long does it generally last?
5. Does the pain ever awaken you from sleep?
6. Is the pain ever so severe that it is unbearable and interferes with your normal daily activities?
7. How would you describe the pain? Cramping, aching, burning, knifelike, or . . . ?
8. Have you found anything you can do or take to alleviate the pain?
9. Does eating or drinking make the pain better or worse?
10. Have you identified certain foods that seem to trigger pain or diarrhea?
11. Describe your typical pattern of bowel movements and the consistency of feces. (For example, one bowel movement, every three days, which is hard and difficult to pass, or two

or three loose, watery bowel movements a day.)

12. Has this pattern remained constant, or has it changed in recent months?

13. Is the pain usually relieved after a bowel movement?

14. Are the bowel movements more loose or more frequent after the onset of pain?

15. Do you have any of the following associated symptoms? (Circle those that apply to you.)
    a. Bloating
    b. Belching
    c. Gas
    d. Nausea
    e. Vomiting

16. Have you lost weight in recent months? If so, how much over what time period?

17. Have you passed blood in your stool or had black, tarry bowel movements?

18. Have you previously been evaluated for these complaints? If so, what tests were performed, and what were the results?

19. Comment on the effectiveness or side effects of any previously prescribed medications that you have taken for your complaints.

PART II

SMOKER: Yes ☐   No ☐
Packs per day _____
For how many years? _____
If a former smoker, when did you quit? _____

ALCOHOL: Yes ☐   No ☐
Drinks per week (average) _____
Have you ever felt guilty about the amount you drink or have you ever felt a need to control your drinking? Yes ☐   No ☐

CAFFEINE: Cups of coffee per day _____
Other (tea, cola, etc.) _____

MEDICATIONS: List medications, prescription and nonprescription, taken regularly. Please include dosage, frequency, and how long you have taken them.

_____

_____

_____

ALLERGIES: List allergies and type of reaction (e.g., penicillin—rash)

_____

_____

_____

_____

Please list those medical problems that your immediate family members have or had. If deceased, list the age and cause of death if known (e.g., father—high blood pressure, deceased age 50—heart attack)

_____

_____

_____

_____

RATE YOUR OVERALL HEALTH
Poor ☐   Fair ☐   Good ☐   Excellent ☐

EXERCISE: Do you exercise regularly? Yes ☐   No ☐
If yes, describe the types of exercise and frequency:

_____

_____

_____

NUTRITION AND DIET:

How many meals do you eat each day? _____

Do you usually eat breakfast? Yes ☐   No ☐

Do you diet frequently and/or are you now dieting? Yes ☐ No ☐

Do you eat, for you, a balanced diet?

Almost always ☐   Sometimes ☐   Rarely ☐

LIST ANY FOOD SUPPLEMENTS OR VITAMINS YOU TAKE REGULARLY:

_____

_____

_____

DO YOU HAVE OR HAVE YOU EVER BEEN TREATED FOR ANY OF THE FOLLOW-ING? Please check yes or no. If you check yes, please give date of treatment or occurrence.

	YES	DATE	NO
Asthma or wheezing	☐	_____	☐
Hayfever or allergies	☐	_____	☐
Tuberculosis	☐	_____	☐
Chronic or persistent cough	☐	_____	☐
Chronic chest condition	☐	_____	☐
Frequent colds, sinus or nose trouble	☐	_____	☐
Stomach or duodenal ulcers	☐	_____	☐
Persistent or recurrent indigestion	☐	_____	☐
Bowel or intestinal trouble	☐	_____	☐
Gallbladder stones or colic	☐	_____	☐
Liver trouble or jaundice	☐	_____	☐
Dysentery or colitis	☐	_____	☐
Rectal trouble or bleeding	☐	_____	☐
Diabetes or sugar in urine	☐	_____	☐
Kidney trouble	☐	_____	☐
High blood pressure or hypertension	☐	_____	☐
Heart trouble, murmurs, or heart attack	☐	_____	☐
Chest pain	☐	_____	☐
Shortness of breath	☐	_____	☐

	Yes	Date	No
Chronic or recurrent eye trouble	☐	_____	☐
Chronic or recurrent ear trouble	☐	_____	☐
Any birth abnormalities	☐	_____	☐
Fatigue	☐	_____	☐
Insomnia	☐	_____	☐
Snoring	☐	_____	☐
Serious bodily injury	☐	_____	☐
Rheumatism or arthritis	☐	_____	☐
Rheumatic fever	☐	_____	☐
Swollen or painful joints	☐	_____	☐
Backache or back injury	☐	_____	☐
Rupture or hernia	☐	_____	☐
Skin disease, rash, or acne	☐	_____	☐
Fainting spells	☐	_____	☐
Stroke	☐	_____	☐
Paralysis	☐	_____	☐
Epilepsy, seizures, convulsions	☐	_____	☐
Varicose veins	☐	_____	☐
Piles or hemorrhoids	☐	_____	☐
Painful or difficult urination	☐	_____	☐
Hypoglycemia	☐	_____	☐
Goiter or thyroid trouble	☐	_____	☐
High metabolism	☐	_____	☐
Low metabolism	☐	_____	☐
Cancer	☐	_____	☐
Anemia	☐	_____	☐
Protein, blood, or pus in urine	☐	_____	☐
Frequent headaches	☐	_____	☐
Migraine headaches	☐	_____	☐
Alcohol addiction	☐	_____	☐
Drug addiction	☐	_____	☐
Sexual problems	☐	_____	☐

HOSPITAL ADMISSIONS FOR: SURGERY, INJURY, OR MATERNITY

Diagnosis   Mo/Year   Hospital/City   Physician

_____

_____

_____

FEMALE PATIENTS ONLY

Menstrual cycles began at age _____
Date of last period _____
Describe any menstrual irregularity:

_____

_____

Total number of pregnancies _____
Total number of miscarriages or abortions _____
Have you gone through menopause? Yes ☐   No ☐
If yes, at what age? _____
Do you take calcium supplements? Yes ☐   No ☐

■

Diet Diary

NAME _____

DATE _____

Time	Food	Amount	Symptoms
____	_____	_____	_____
____	_____	_____	_____
____	_____	_____	_____
____	_____	_____	_____
____	_____	_____	_____
____	_____	_____	_____
____	_____	_____	_____
____	_____	_____	_____
____	_____	_____	_____
____	_____	_____	_____
____	_____	_____	_____
____	_____	_____	_____
____	_____	_____	_____
____	_____	_____	_____
____	_____	_____	_____
____	_____	_____	_____

Stress Level: 1   2   3   4   5   (low - high)

Exercise:

APPENDIX 2

COMMON QUESTIONS AND ANSWERS ABOUT IBS

Question: What causes IBS?

Answer: Although the exact cause of IBS is not known, there seems to exist an underlying abnormality that results in the disruption of normal rhythmic contractions of the intestinal tract. Abdominal pain and altered bowel function (variations of diarrhea or constipation) are the symptoms experienced when intestinal contractions are disrupted. Emotional stress and certain foods lead the list of factors that may trigger symptoms. Genetic predisposition as well as recurrent abdominal pains during childhood may predispose one to the development of this disorder.

> PATIENTS' HINT:
>
> *Always have "safe" foods on hand whether at home or traveling.*

Question: How is the diagnosis of IBS established?

Answer: Unfortunately, there is no conclusive test to firmly establish a diagnosis of IBS. The diagnosis is suspected when the physician elicits characteristic symptoms during a medical history. Physical examination, blood tests, stool specimens, X rays, and endoscopy may be employed to evaluate for other conditions that may mimic IBS or coexist with it.

PATIENTS' HINT:

Avoid tight-fitting garments.

Question: How is IBS treated?

Answer: Treatment begins with patient education. It is important to develop an understanding of what is and what is not known about IBS and the underlying intestinal rhythmic disorder. Appropriate lifestyle changes such as dietary changes, stress reduction, and exercise should be made. Appropriate remedies or medications may be prescribed to treat certain aspects of the disorder. Ideally, a cooperative team approach will be developed with your physician to help you gain control over your IBS symptoms.

PATIENTS' HINT:

Frequent small meals are better than one or two large meals.

Question: Is there a cure for IBS?

Answer: There is as yet no cure for IBS in the same sense that a course of antibiotics may cure an infection. IBS will often cause periodic symptoms, with symptom-free intervals lasting days, months, or years. However, you can learn to gain control over your symptoms, thereby increasing the symptom-free intervals. To the extent that you are able to remain symptom free by following and refining the suggestions outlined in this book, you may actually experience a "cure."

PATIENTS' HINT:

Remember, foods with a high fat content are a common trigger of negative symptoms.

Question: What is the difference between colitis and IBS?

Answer: The term "colitis" implies inflammation of the colon. IBS is not associated with colon inflammation and should not be confused with inflammatory bowel disease (IBD). IBD sufferers will often have bloody diarrhea, fever, and weight loss—symptoms associated with colon inflammation.

PATIENTS' HINT:

Start low and go slow when increasing dietary fiber. Take your fiber supplements around mealtime.

Question: Will IBS predispose me to more serious disorders?

Answer: No, having IBS will not make you more likely to develop such conditions as inflammatory bowel disease, colon cancer, or colon polyps. And IBS will not require surgery. At the same time, managing your IBS well will not protect you from developing other bowel conditions, and if you see any change in your usual pattern of symptoms, you should consult your physician.

PATIENTS' HINT:

Establish a consistent time for elimination.

Question: What are the warning signs that something other than IBS is going on?

Answer: A partial listing of worrisome symptoms includes fever, weight loss, painful or difficult swallowing, persistent vomiting, a sense of feeling full sooner than usual during meals, new or different pains, a change in bowel pattern—particularly worsening constipation, narrower stools, or blood in the bowel movement. If any of these symptoms occur, contact your doctor.

PATIENTS' HINT:

Take a walk to relieve gas, or bring your knees up forward to your chest a few times.

Question: Are there tests for lactose intolerance?

Answer: Yes, the hydrogen breath test is a simple, effective test, usually conducted at the GI lab of a hospital, to determine an inability to completely digest the sugar lactose found in dairy products. The test, which takes two to three hours, involves ingestion of lactose and the periodic analysis of expired air. If lactose is not completely digested and absorbed in the intestinal tract, it will eventually end up in the colon, where it will be fermented by colonic bacteria. During this process, above-normal amounts of hydrogen gas are produced, some of which is absorbed into the bloodstream and later expired through the lungs.

PATIENTS' HINT:

Map out exits with rest room facilities when taking a highway trip.

Question: Should I take calcium supplements if I have a lactose intolerance?

Answer: If you have a lactose intolerance and for this reason avoid dairy products, you should take calcium supplements. You should take between 1000 and 1500 milligrams of calcium daily.

Alternatively, persons with lactose intolerance may tolerate dairy products by taking lactase enzyme supplements when they are eating dairy products.

PATIENTS' HINT:

Take care not to swallow air while eating or drinking.

Question: Do spicy foods make IBS symptoms worse?

Answer: Spicy foods sometimes make IBS symptoms worse but not always. For example, many patients have told me they cannot tolerate Mexican food because it is "too spicy." Further investigation has revealed it was the high fat content of the average Mexican meal (fried chips, cheese, refried beans, sour cream, guacamole) rather than the hot, spicy salsa that triggered the symptoms. These patients can enjoy modified Mexican, Cajun, and similar entrées that have reduced fat but retain their distinctive spices.

PATIENTS' HINT:

Check whether adjusting your posture and stretching tall reduces pain in the abdomen.

Question: Is there a relationship between IBS and sexual dysfunction?

Answer: One study suggests that women with IBS are more likely to complain of uncomfortable intercourse than women with peptic ulcer disease. The explanation for this finding might be that abdominal cramps, gas, and bloating make intercourse less pleasurable and thus lessen sexual gratification. Many women have reported enhanced sexuality with mastery and control of their IBS symptoms.

PATIENTS' HINT:

While lying down, clockwise self-massage with one hand applied to the abdominal wall may help relieve discomfort. Some people find that warmth applied to the abdomen relieves symptoms.

Question: Are herbs useful for treating IBS symptoms?

Answer: Unfortunately, there is a dearth of scientific information about the use of herbs to treat intestinal disorders. That is not to say herbs are ineffective; it is only a sad commentary on the fact that the medical community has not been active in pursuing natural remedies. One exception is peppermint oil, which has been studied and appears to be a natural antispasmodic if taken in the correct dose. In fact, many IBS sufferers find caffeine-free peppermint tea quite effective in relieving abdominal cramps. I cannot make a firm recommendation regarding the use of herbs to treat IBS at this time, but I have worked with patients who have found various herbal preparations useful.

PATIENTS' HINT:

Check if extremities are chilled, as this may trigger negative symptoms.

APPENDIX 3

—◾—

ALL ABOUT MEDICATION

This appendix contains detailed information about the various types of medications that may be used to treat IBS. The information is organized by therapeutic category and class of medications. This appendix is intended to supplement, but not replace, information provided by your physician and the drug manufacturer. This is not an exhaustive list of all medications of possible benefit in treating IBS, but rather a list of those medications that have shown possible benefit in my own experience or in clinical studies. For ease of recognition, we have included a listing of the more commonly prescribed trade and generic names in each class.

Remember that any medication is capable of producing side effects. Rare individual or so-called "idiosyncratic" reactions may occur in susceptible people. The likelihood that anyone will experience a side effect may relate to the dose or duration of therapy. Concomitant use of other medications may increase the likelihood of experiencing an unwanted drug interaction or side effect.

The use of medications (whether prescription or not) during pregnancy may pose risks to the developing fetus as well as the mother. Contact your doctor regarding the use of any medication if you are pregnant or if you are breast-feeding.

Antispasmodics

COMMON EXAMPLES

Clidinium bromide (Quarzan), dicyclomine (Bentyl), hyoscyamine sulfate (Anaspaz, Cystospaz, Cystospaz-M, Levsin, Levsinex Timecaps).

Note: Combination preparations containing an antispasmodic and various other agents are also available. Phenobarbital, hyoscyamine sulfate, atropine sulfate and hyoscine hydrobromide (Donnatal), chlordiazepoxide hydrochloride, and clidinium bromide (Librax).

GENERAL INFORMATION

The antispasmodics work by reducing spasms of the stomach and intestines. These drugs inhibit the action of nerves that regulate the intestinal smooth muscle and certain secretory glands found in the intestinal tract. Antispasmodics may be helpful for treating symptoms associated with irritable bowel syndrome, peptic ulcer disease, diarrhea, and diverticulosis.

POSSIBLE SIDE EFFECTS

Difficulty in urination, blurred vision, nausea, vomiting, bloating, constipation, nervousness, anxiety, delirium, drowsiness, insomnia, rapid heartbeat, nasal congestion, rash, itching, flushing, decreased sweating (which may predispose one to heat exhaustion), and impotence.

HOW TO USE THE MEDICATION

Antispasmodics are best taken 30 minutes before meals. Since they may cause drowsiness, caution should be used when performing tasks that require alertness. Notify your doctor if you develop any of the above-mentioned side effects, the most common of which are dry mouth, difficulty in urination, constipation, and increased sensitivity to light. Patients with glaucoma should not use antispasmodics. Eye pain may be a side effect in persons with previously undiagnosed glaucoma.

Drugs Used to Treat Diarrhea

COMMON EXAMPLES

Bismuth subsalicylate (Pepto-Bismol), camphorated tincture of opium (Paregoric), cholestyramine (Questran), colestipol (Colestid), diphenoxylate hydrochloride and atropine sulfate (Lomotil), kaolin and pectin (Kaopectate), kaolin pectin, hyoscyamine sulfate, atropine sulfate and scopolamine hydrobromide (Donnagel), loperamide hydrochloride (Imodium).

GENERAL INFORMATION

Diarrhea may be defined as stools that are more frequent than usual (generally more often than three times a day) or stools that are excessively liquid. There are various causes of diarrhea, including diarrhea associated with IBS. The various antidiarrheal agents have different mechanisms of action. Caution should be used when treating diarrhea associated with infections of the gastrointestinal tract, since antidiarrheal drugs may interfere with the body's attempt to get rid of the infectious agent.

The antispasmodics have been used as antidiarrheal agents, but their primary effect is to relieve cramps by reducing intestinal smooth-muscle contractions. The opioids (Imodium, Lomotil, Paregoric) are probably the most effective, prompt-acting antidiarrheal agents. They act by slowing gastrointestinal motility and prolonging the transit time of the intestinal contents to allow more time for absorption of water and electrolytes.

Other agents used to treat diarrhea include the antisecretory agents (Pepto-Bismol). These agents help stimulate absorption of fluids and electrolytes across the intestinal wall. The so-called "adsorbents" (Kaopectate) are thought to act by adsorbing excess water in the gastrointestinal tract. The so-called "bile-acid sequestrants" (Colestid, Questran) relieve diarrhea that is thought to be secondary to excessive bile salts (which are produced by the liver). These agents may be particularly effective in individuals with diarrhea after having gallbladder removal (cholecystectomy).

Side effects vary with the different classes of antidiarrheal agents. All of these agents may cause constipation as a side effect and should not be used when diarrhea is associated with blood in the bowel movement or with fever.

In addition to causing constipation, the opioids may cause nausea, vomiting, drowsiness, dizziness, nervousness, confusion, blurred vision, dry mouth, difficulty urinating, and an irregular heartbeat.

Bismuth subsalicylate may cause dark stools or a dark tongue. The adsorbents are generally quite safe but may interfere with the adsorption of other medications. A two- to three-hour interval is recommended between the administration of adsorbents and the administration of other drugs.

HOW TO USE THE MEDICATION
Your physician will need to determine the appropriate antidiarrheal agent for you to use. Antidiarrheal agents are most helpful when access to a bathroom is limited and before anxiety-producing situations such as a job interview if diarrhea is anticipated.

Drugs Used to Treat Constipation

COMMON EXAMPLES
Bulk-forming agents—methylcellulose (Citrucel), polycarbophil (Equalactin, Fibercon, Mitrolan), psyllium (Fiberall, Hydrocil, Konsyl, Metamucil, Perdiem).

Mineral oil—(Agoral plain, Kondremul, Milkinol).

Lactulose—(Cephulac, Chronulac, Duphulac).

GENERAL INFORMATION
The normal bowel movement should be neither hard nor loose and should be easily passed without straining. Constipation occurs when the stools are hard and difficult to pass. Therefore, the consistency of the stool rather than the frequency of elimina-

tion determines the extent of constipation. Laxatives are frequently misused because of lack of understanding of bowel function. For example, when potent laxatives are taken, the colon may empty of all fecal material, and two or three days may be required to re-establish a sufficient quantity of fecal mass for the next bowel movement. This lag time may be perceived as constipation and more laxatives may be ingested, resulting in a vicious cycle.

In most instances, adequate intake of fruits, vegetables, and grains in an active individual will help maintain normal stool frequency and consistency. If these measures fail, it may become necessary to take soaked natural psyllium, bulk-forming agents, or an occasional laxative. The bulk-forming agents are most frequently prescribed for IBS sufferers to "normalize" the bowel movements. The bulk agents work by retaining water and will make a hard stool softer. Although traditionally thought to be most helpful for constipation, they also may be of benefit in treating diarrhea by absorbing the excess water in the gut and thus making the stool firmer.

Mineral oil works as a lubricant, softening the feces and allowing for easier passage of a hard stool. It may be useful for the short-term treatment of constipation.

Lactulose may be effective for treating people with constipation-predominant IBS if other measures fail. Lactulose, which is a sugar containing lactose and galactose, works by drawing water and electrolytes into the colon, making the stool softer. Because of its colon-specific site of action, lactulose avoids many of the potentially harmful effects that result from the absorption of many laxatives.

So-called "contact" and "stimulant" laxatives are widely used and abused. It is best to avoid using them regularly.

POSSIBLE SIDE EFFECTS

Bulk-forming agents are usually safe when taken with adequate amounts of liquid (at least eight ounces per dose). Intestinal obstruction may occur if adequate amounts of liquid are not taken.

Rare allergic reactions to psyllium products have been reported.

Excessive use of mineral oil may interfere with absorption of fat-soluble vitamins (A, D, E, K). Mineral oil may inadvertently be aspirated into the lungs, producing a chemical pneumonia (lipid pneumonia). This complication may be prevented by avoiding the recumbent position for at least two hours after taking the mineral oil.

The initial administration of lactulose for treatment of constipation may cause excessive gas and cramps, particularly in individuals with coexisting lactose intolerance. These symptoms often improve with continued use and the establishment of regular soft bowel movements. Excessive doses may produce watery stools.

How to Use the Medication

Remember to take bulk-forming agents with adequate amounts of liquid, preferably around mealtime, so that they mix with the food. If you are overweight, take them before meals to help curb your appetite. If you are at or below your ideal body weight, take them after meals. Be patient—it may take up to 72 hours for the initial laxative effects to be noted.

Mineral oil is most effective if taken on an empty stomach. Be sure to take it with a full glass of liquid. Mineral oil may leak from the rectum, causing soiling of the undergarments.

Lactulose may be mixed with fruit juice or water to improve the taste. Remember, gas and cramps may occur with the initial doses. Start with a low dose and gradually increase every few days as needed.

Drugs Used to Reduce Gas

Common Examples

Charcoal (Charcoal, Charcocaps), simethicone (Gas-X, Extra Strength Gas-X, Mylicon, Mylicon-80, Phazyme, Phazyme-95, Phazyme-125, and Silain), simethicone and charcoal (Charcoal

169

Plus). Various other combinations with antispasmodics and antacids or digestive enzymes are available.

Too much gas in the gastrointestinal tract may cause cramps, belching, bloating, and flatulence. Persons with IBS have been shown to be sensitive to "normal" amounts of intestinal gas. Air swallowing, or aerophagia, is one means by which excessive amounts of gas enter the intestinal tract. Avoiding carbonated beverages, gum and mints (which both promote the swallowing of air), and gas-producing foods (such as beans and certain fruits and vegetables) will help to decrease gastrointestinal gas. If these measures fail, there are various products that reduce gaseous distension.

Simethicone has an antifoaming action that is purported to help small, mucus-surrounded gas bubbles aggregate into larger units that may be more easily eliminated by belching or passing flatus. Simethicone is designed to minimize gas formation and relieve entrapped gas in the gastrointestinal tract.

Gas that accumulates in the gastrointestinal tract may be adsorbed by charcoal. The gas-charcoal mixture is then eliminated from the body at the time of defecation. Because of charcoal's adsorption properties, it is often used in various filtering devices, such as water purification systems. It is also frequently used to bind drugs ingested during an accidental or intentional drug overdose.

The evidence suggesting that simethicone and charcoal preparations reduce symptoms of intestinal gas is inconclusive. In my experience, however, some people find these agents useful.

POSSIBLE SIDE EFFECTS

Simethicone appears to be very safe. No adverse reactions to simethicone have been reported, but like other medications, it should be avoided in cases of known sensitivity to any ingredient found in the formulation. Charcoal binds medications and may reduce their effectiveness. Charcoal will turn the stool black.

Simethicone should be taken at meals and at bedtime. Chew the chewable tablets thoroughly before swallowing. Ideally, charcoal should be taken after meals. Take two hours before or one hour after taking other drugs (including birth control pills) to prevent interference of drug absorption.

Anti-Ulcer Agents

COMMON EXAMPLES
H_2 Antagonists—cimetidine (Tagamet), famotidine (Pepcid), nizatidine (Axid), ranitidine (Zantac).

Miscellaneous agents—omeprazole (Losec), sucralfate (Carafate).

GENERAL INFORMATION
Although not indicated specifically for treatment of IBS, the anti-ulcer agents are frequently prescribed (often inappropriately) on a trial basis to treat persons with various abdominal complaints. They are used to treat upper abdominal "burning" pains (dyspepsia), whether or not a definite ulcer of the stomach or duodenum (peptic ulcer disease) is present. "Nonulcer dyspepsia" is the term used when burning pains located in the upper abdomen exist and no frank ulceration is shown by upper gastrointestinal X rays or direct observation by endoscopy.

I am not suggesting that there is an association between IBS and peptic ulcer disease or nonulcer dyspepsia, but many of the IBS sufferers I encounter in my practice have at some time been treated with one of the anti-ulcer agents. This treatment has often been attempted to alleviate vague, burning abdominal complaints or simply out of frustration when other measures to control IBS symptoms have failed. The H_2 receptor antagonists are the most frequently prescribed agents for peptic ulcer disease and have for the most part replaced the use of over-the-counter

171

antacids (Di-Gel, Gaviscon, Maalox, Mylanta) for this disorder. The H_2 receptor is a histamine receptor found in the stomach; when blocked, it decreases stomach acid secretion. This blockage of stomach acid secretion is thought to promote healing of ulcerations in the stomach and duodenum.

Omeprazole is a new class of stomach acid inhibitors that is thought to directly block the acid pump located in specialized cells lining the stomach. Omeprazole is at least as effective as the H_2 antagonists, if not more so, in treating peptic ulcer disease. There is concern about the safety of this agent with extended use, and results of long-term clinical studies are not yet available. For this reason, omeprazole is reserved for special disorders of stomach acid hypersecretion and when more traditional medications (antacids, H_2 antagonists, sucralfate) have failed.

Sucralfate is another effective agent for treatment of peptic ulcer disease. Sucralfate appears to act by physically coating ulcers and thus serving as a barrier to help prevent further damage by stomach acid.

POSSIBLE SIDE EFFECTS

The overall incidence of adverse reactions to the H_2 antagonists is low. Possible side effects include diarrhea, headache, dizziness, muscle aches, rash, and confusion (particularly in the elderly). Since these agents may interact with other drugs, notify your doctor if you are taking any other medication (whether prescription or not) in addition to the H_2 antagonist.

Few adverse reactions have been noted with omeprazole, but since it is a relatively new drug, experience with it is limited.

Sucralfate is not significantly absorbed, and consequently has very few side effects. Constipation and other minor gastrointestinal disturbances occur infrequently.

HOW TO USE THE MEDICATION

Anti-ulcer agents should be taken only under the direction of your physician. Notify your doctor of any other medications you are taking to avoid drug interactions. If you are taking antacids as well as H_2 antagonists, do not take them at the same time (allow one hour between the two). Carafate should be taken one hour before meals and at bedtime.

Prokinetic Agents

COMMON EXAMPLES

Metoclopramide (Octamide, Reglan).

GENERAL INFORMATION

The prokinetic agents actually increase motility of the intestinal tract—particularly the stomach and small intestine. They are most frequently used to treat disorders such as reflux esophagitis (acid indigestion) and gastroparesis (delayed emptying of the stomach—commonly seen in diabetics). I have occasionally found these agents helpful in treating the upper abdominal bloating and nausea seen in some IBS sufferers, particularly when constipation is present.

POSSIBLE SIDE EFFECTS

Metoclopramide may infrequently induce nausea, diarrhea, and abdominal cramps. Drowsiness, anxiety, dizziness, insomnia, headache, and depression are other potential side effects that are likely mediated through reactions of this medication in the nervous system. Spontaneous flow of breast milk, breast tenderness, and gynecomastia (breast enlargement in males) are occasionally seen.

With long-term use, symptoms of Parkinson's disease may develop—tremor, muscle rigidity, and general slowing of muscular activity (bradykinesia).

HOW TO USE THE MEDICATION

Metoclopramide should only be taken at the advice and under the direction of a physician. Ideally, the medication should be taken 30 minutes before meals and at bedtime.

Digestive Enzymes

Common examples—pancreatin (Creon, Pancreatin), pancrease (Cotazym, Cotazym-S, Entolase, Festal II, Ku-Zyme, Pancrease, Zymase).

GENERAL INFORMATION

Adequate production of the enzymes lipase, protease, and amylase by the pancreas allow for optimum digestion of fat, protein, and carbohydrate. If there is an established pancreatic insufficiency—as seen with cystic fibrosis, with chronic pancreatitis (chronic inflammation of the pancreas), and after pancreatectomy (surgical removal of the pancreas)—treatment with digestive enzymes may be necessary. These agents have been promoted as "digestive aids" for the treatment of a variety of digestive disorders, including IBS.

POSSIBLE SIDE EFFECTS

Because the enzymes are derived from pork pancreas glands, individuals sensitive to pork should avoid them. Inadvertent inhalation of powdered preparations may precipitate an asthma attack.

HOW TO USE THE MEDICATION

Digestive enzymes should be taken immediately before or with meals. The powder may be irritating to the skin or lungs if spilled or inhaled. Do not crush or chew capsules or tablets.

Anti-Anxiety Agents

COMMON EXAMPLES

Benzodiazepines—alprazolam (Xanax), chlordiazepoxide (Librium), clonazepam (Klonopin), chlorazepate dipotassium (Tranxene), diazepam (Valium), lorazepam (Ativan), oxazepam (Serax), prazepam (Centrax). Nonbenzodizepine agents—buspirone (Buspar).

GENERAL INFORMATION

As the name implies, anti-anxiety agents are used in the treatment of generalized anxiety (nervousness) disorders. In recent years, much attention has been focused on the use or overuse of these drugs. I favor the use of relaxation techniques (which must be learned and practiced) over the use of medications to treat anxiety. However, these agents may be useful in treating symptoms of IBS that are clearly exacerbated by stressful situations—for example, "nervous diarrhea," which some authorities believe should be considered a separate condition from IBS.

The benzodiazepines are ideally suited for short-term, intermittent treatment of anxiety and associated physical symptoms that might interfere with normal daily function. Short-term, intermittent use prevents many of the problems associated with chronic use of benzodiazepines, such as physical and psychological dependency. If physical dependency (addiction or habituation) occurs, abrupt withdrawal of the medication will result in rebound worsening of the anxiety symptoms as well as rapid heart rate, tremor, increased blood pressure, and sweating. Psychological dependency—subjective dependency without associated physical symptoms such as rapid heart rate, elevated blood pressure, and sweating—may occur with any medication. Psychiatric consultation may be advised for those persons in need of chronic therapy.

Buspirone is a relatively new, nonbenzodiazepine anti-anxiety agent that causes less sedation and is unlikely to produce withdrawal symptoms associated with physical dependency. For this reason, it may be more appropriate for the treatment of chronic anxiety. The anti-anxiety effect will gradually occur over one to four weeks. This gradual onset of action makes buspirone unsuited for brief, intermittent therapy. For that type of therapy, benzodiazepines would be more appropriate. Studies evaluating buspirone for treatment of IBS and premenstrual syndrome show some promise.

POSSIBLE SIDE EFFECTS

The most common side effects of the benzodiazepines include sedation, lethargy, and mental clouding. Other, less common side effects include: delirium, vivid dreams, dizziness, depression, blurred vision, headache, low blood pressure, urinary retention or inability to hold urine, and constipation. As mentioned above, long-term use may result in physical and psychological dependency.

Possible adverse reactions to buspirone include: nervousness, headache, weakness, dizziness, depression or excitement, rapid heart rate, tingling sensations of the extremities, sweating, dry mouth, nausea, and diarrhea.

HOW TO USE THE MEDICATION

Benzodiazepines have been shown to have possible adverse effects on the fetus, and should not be taken if you are pregnant or breast-feeding. Like other prescription medications, these agents should always be taken under the direction of your physician and only as prescribed. Use with caution when driving or performing any task that requires mental alertness. Use with alcohol should be avoided, as an additive effect may occur, causing drowsiness. After long-term use, abrupt cessation may result in withdrawal symptoms—worsening anxiety, sweating, rapid heart rate, and increased blood pressure.

Buspirone should also be used with caution when you are driving or performing other tasks that require mental alertness. Avoid use with alcohol. Allow three to four weeks for the maximum anti-anxiety effect to be noted. Some benefit may be obtained after the first week.

Antidepressants

COMMON EXAMPLES

Tricyclic antidepressants—amitriptyline (Elavil, Endep), amoxapine (Asendin), desipramine (Norpramin, Pertofrane), doxepin (Adapin, Sinequan), imipramine (Tofranil), nortriptyline (Aventyl, Pamelor), protriptyline (Vivactyl), and trimipramine (Surmontil).

Miscellaneous antidepressants—bupropion (Wellbutrin), fluoxetine (Prozac), trazodone (Desyrel), alprazolam (Xanax).

GENERAL INFORMATION

Numerous studies have attempted to establish a link between IBS and various psychiatric illnesses, including depression. To date, no single psychological profile has been established in IBS sufferers. Does depression lead to IBS, or do IBS sufferers become depressed as a result of their digestive disorder? Given the complexity of symptoms associated with IBS and the variability of factors that may adversely affect the digestive tract, these questions may never be conclusively answered.

Research suggests that certain subsets of patients with IBS are found to be clinically depressed when evaluated psychologically and that IBS symptoms may improve with treatment of the underlying depressive disorder. Symptoms of depression may include: lack of self-esteem, disturbed sleep patterns, fatigue, decreased appetite, mental clouding, and feeling "blue."

Certain antidepressants also possess anti-anxiety properties and may be helpful in treating symptoms of IBS provoked by stress. Antidepressants have shown benefit in the treatment of various chronic pain syndromes (such as low back pain, headache, fibromyalgia syndrome) and may be helpful for the chronic, recurrent abdominal pain associated with IBS. Through mechanisms that are not clearly understood, it may turn out that antidepressants favorably affect the enteric nervous system (the nerves that control the digestive tract) in IBS sufferers. However they work, antidepressants are occasionally useful as part of the total treatment program for IBS. Most antidepressants take about two to three weeks to achieve their maximum beneficial effect at any given dose. Usually therapy is begun with low doses and gradually increased every two to three weeks as needed.

POSSIBLE SIDE EFFECTS

The tricyclics are the oldest, most established class of antidepressant medication. Common side effects include dry mouth, sedation, and a hung-over feeling. These side effects usually abate with continued use. Other, less common side effects include: sleep disturbance, nightmares, sweating, blurred vision, constipation, rapid heart rate, decreased blood pressure, worsening of glaucoma, and urinary retention. Increased appetite and weight gain may occur with certain tricyclics. With long-term use, symptoms of Parkinson's disease may develop—tremor, muscle rigidity, and general slowing of muscular activity (bradykinesia). These symptoms may become apparent with abrupt withdrawal of the medication.

Check with your physician or pharmacist regarding potential side effects of the miscellaneous antidepressant medications.

HOW TO USE THE MEDICATION

Like other prescription medications, antidepressants must be taken exactly as prescribed. Allow two to three weeks before deciding whether or not they are helping. Exercise caution while driving or performing tasks that require mental alertness. Use with alcohol should be avoided, since sedation will be worsened. Dry mouth and sedation will often lessen with continued use.

Miscellaneous Medications

COMMON EXAMPLES

Calcium channel blockers—diltiazem (Cardizem, Cardizem SR), nicardipine (Cardene), nifedipine (Adalat, Procardia, Procardia XL), nimodipine (Nimotop), verapamil (Calan, Calan SR, Isoptin, Isoptin SR, Verelan).

Nitrogylcerin—*Note:* There are numerous nitroglycerin preparations available. Many are available in generic form, including tablets, capsules, and patches.

Beta blockers—acebutolol (Sectral), atenolol (Tenormin),

Betaxolol (Kerlone), Metoprolol (Lopressor), nadolol (Corgard), penbutolol (Levatol), pindolol (Visken), propranolol (Inderal, Inderal LA), timolol (Blocadren).

GENERAL INFORMATION

The miscellaneous medications listed in this section have been most widely used in the past for treatment of conditions affecting the heart, such as hypertension and angina. There are some studies and case reports available regarding the use of these medications for treatment of IBS and other digestive disorders.

Certain of the calcium channel blockers (such as nifedipine) have been used to treat spasms of the esophagus, which some authorities believe is a variant of IBS. I find verapamil helpful for some IBS sufferers whose predominant symptoms are diarrhea and cramps. Nitroglycerin preparations have also been used to treat esophageal spasm and may be helpful for intestinal cramps. A few reports indicate that certain beta blockers may be of possible benefit in treating symptoms of IBS.

The agents listed in this section are useful for treating a combination of problems, such as hypertension and IBS, or angina and IBS. It is to be hoped that the role of calcium channel blockers, nitroglycerin preparations, and beta blockers in treating IBS will become more evident as more information becomes available.

POSSIBLE SIDE EFFECTS/HOW TO USE THE MEDICATION

Consult your physician or pharmacist regarding possible side effects if one of these medications is prescribed. How to use the medication will vary greatly, depending on which medication is prescribed and for what aspects of IBS.

LACTOSE-FREE DIET

Remember that lactose intolerance or sensitivity, like many other food intolerances and sensitivities, is quantitative as well as qualitative. Most lactose-intolerant individuals become symptomatic (experiencing gas, cramps, bloating, and diarrhea) after ingesting 12 grams of lactose. This is the approximate content of an 8-ounce glass of milk. Some people, particularly those with IBS and lactose intolerance, may become symptomatic after as little as 3 grams of lactose. Lactose may be better tolerated when taken with other foods. Small amounts of butter and cheese may be tolerated, depending on the individual.

Read labels carefully! Avoid any product that contains milk, milk products, milk solids, whey, casein, curd, lactose, or galactose. Small amounts of these substances may be tolerated; however, the quantity of lactose may not be stated on the label.

Lactase enzyme supplements may be used to treat milk to decrease the lactose content or may be taken with milk or lactose-containing products. Lactase-treated milk is sweeter than regular milk.

Lactose-intolerant individuals who avoid all dairy products should take calcium supplements. Usually 1000 to 1500 milligrams of elemental calcium should be taken daily.

Following is a comprehensive listing of common foods to

avoid and those that are allowed, depending on the severity of your lactose intolerance.

LACTOSE-FREE DIET

Type of Food	Foods Allowed	Foods to Avoid
Milk or milk products	Nondairy products that do not contain lactose. Soybean milk may be used as a substitute.	All milk or milk products as listed on the previous page. For example: yogurt, cheese, ice cream, sherbet.
Eggs	All.	None.
Vegetables	All (organic vegetables are preferable where available).	Vegetables prepared with foods to avoid such as cream, margarine, butter.
Meat, fish, poultry	All types of meat, fish, and poultry that are not creamed or breaded.	Creamed or breaded meat, fish, or poultry. Luncheon meats, sausage, and any processed meat that contains milk products.
Bread, grains, and cereals	All products that do not contain milk or milk products.	All products containing milk or milk products.
Fats	All types of fats that do not contain milk or milk products.	Butter, margarine, sour cream, or any product that contains milk or milk products.

Type of Food	Foods Allowed	Foods to Avoid
Soups	Those broth-based soups that do not contain milk or milk products.	Cream soups or any soups that contain milk or milk products.
Fruits and fruit juices	All fresh, frozen, or canned products without lactose (organic fruit preferable where available).	Any product prepared with lactose.
Desserts	Angel food cake, Jell-O, sorbets, or any product made without milk products.	Most commercial desserts and any product made with milk or milk products.
Miscellaneous	Nuts, peanut butter, pure sugar, and honey.	All gravies, sauces, candies, liqueurs, or commercial mixers made with milk or milk products, molasses.

FOODS HIGH IN FIBER

This list gives the approximate fiber content of some common high-fiber foods. Use it as a guide to familiarize yourself with foods to include in your diet to achieve the desired intake of 30 to 40 grams of dietary fiber. Remember to increase your intake of dietary fiber gradually so that your intestinal tract can adjust, preventing excessive gas and bloating.

Food Source	*Dietary Fiber (grams)*
GRAINS AND BREAKFAST CEREALS	
Corn Flakes, 3/4 cup	2.0
Puffed Wheat, 3/4 cup	1.4
Raisin Bran, 3/4 cup	1.0
Shredded Wheat, 1 large biscuit	2.7
Rice, 1/2 cup cooked brown	2.4
Rice, 1/2 cup cooked white	0.1
FRUITS	
Apple, 1 medium	2.8
Banana, 1 medium	1.8
Berries, 1/2 cup	2.0
Cherries, 15 large	1.0
Figs, 2 dried, small	6.4
Grapes, 16	2.0
Orange, 1 medium	3.2
Peach, 1 medium	2.2
Pineapple, 3/4 cup	0.5
Plums, 2 medium	1.5
Prunes, 8 large	2.0
Strawberries, 10 large	2.0

Food Source	Dietary Fiber (grams)
NUTS	
Brazil nuts, 1/4 cup	2.5
Filberts, 1/4 cup	5.0
Peanuts, 1/4 cup	3.3
Sunflower seeds, 1/4 cup	4.0
BREADS AND CRACKERS	
Rye crackers, 6	2.0
Rye bread, 1 slice	1.0
White bread, 1 slice	0.5
Whole wheat bread, 1 slice	1.4
VEGETABLES	
Asparagus, 3/4 cup	3.1
Baked beans, 1/3 cup	6.0
Beans, 1/2 cup pinto	5.3
Beans, 1/2 cup white	5.0
Beans, 1/2 cup green	2.1
Beans, 1/2 cup kidney	5.8
Beets, 1/2 cup	2.5
Broccoli tops, 1/2 cup	3.0
Brussels sprouts, 1/2 cup	2.8
Cabbage, 1/2 cup	2.8
Cauliflower, 1/2 cup	1.8
Lettuce, 1/2 cup	0.5
Onion, 1/2 cup	2.1
Carrots, 1/2 cup	3.0
Peas, 1/2 cup	5.0
Popcorn, 1 cup popped	0.5
Potato, 1 med. baked	3.0
Spinach, 1/2 cup boiled	5.7
Tomatoes, 1 small	1.4
Turnips, 2/3 cup	2.0
Sweet Corn, 1/2 cup	4.7
Zucchini squash, 1/2 cup	2.7

APPENDIX 6

HOW TO STOP SMOKING

Cigarette smoking is the greatest single cause of chronic ill-ness, disability, and death in North America. The simple fact is that YOU CAN QUIT.

Cigarette smoking threatens a smoker's survival, decreases energy levels, increases risk of heart disease, lung disease, and cancer, and decreases his or her ability to fight infection. Secondhand smoke also threatens a smoker's spouse, children, coworkers, and friends.

Now that the U.S. surgeon general has declared nicotine an "addictive" drug, you can count on an increased number of quick cures and products for those seeking to quit. In fact, there are numerous programs and products with little proven success, de-signed primarily to separate you from your money. The unfortu-nate fact is that there is no simple, quick, or easy route to perma-nent independence of tobacco. To successfully quit smoking, you must be aware of two aspects of your habits: your associative habits and your dependence on nicotine.

Associative habits are those you have developed over the years. Smoking is particularly satisfying with coffee, after a meal, first thing in the morning, with a drink in the evening, and so on. Many smokers overcome this habit by waiting for a short period after the associative activity before smoking a cigarette. For example, have the cup of coffee, wait half an hour, then have the cigarette. If you're one of those who reach for that pack as soon as they rise, then get up, wait a half hour, then have your first cigarette. The secret is to break up these associative habits, whatever they are. Do one activity, then the other.

To overcome a dependence on nicotine, seek brands with increasingly lower nicotine content. Most brands that are lower in tars and nicotine list their comparative contents, either on the package or in their advertisements. This should be a well-thought-out process so that you know what brand you will be going to next. Do not go to the lowest nicotine all at once; to be successful, you need a gradual withdrawal of your dependence.

Some people prefer to quit cold turkey. This technique is often effective but may increase the intensity of nicotine withdrawal symptoms—namely, irritability and anxiety. An advantage to this approach, however, is that the entire process is shortened. I encourage my patients who have had to quit for various reasons, such as an illness requiring hospitalization, to not resume the habit, since they have already gone through the withdrawal period.

Some authorities insist it is best to set a target date for quitting, say, six months away, or 18 weeks away. Then tell everyone about that date. ("On September 25, I will stop smoking.") Others find setting a date an additional stress. Remember, you are seeking to achieve something permanently beneficial to your health. If you have been smoking for several years, the few weeks or months you devote to a concerted effort to quit are well worth the struggle. You emerge a winner.

Seek the advice of your physician. New practices or methods may be available that are well worth exploring.

There are a number of professionally run clinics and groups sponsored by medical centers and hospitals. Perhaps there are several in your area. You may want to join them for their support and suggestions. The American Cancer Society has a wealth of information and some sound policies and practices for those who want to quit smoking. Contact and support your local branch.

After you have made up your mind to quit, try to maintain as nearly a normal schedule as possible and avoid stressful situations whenever possible while attempting to quit.

What if you fail? Many smokers have failed in their first attempts to quit. Do not be discouraged. Studies indicate that with repeated attempts, the probability of success actually increases.

Don't worry about gaining weight. Perhaps you'll gain 10 to 15 pounds, mainly because food tastes better and you enjoy the oral gratification achieved through eating rather than smoking. But weight is much easier to deal with than smoking, and as a nonsmoker, you will learn to relish more healthful snacks and discover increased energy through exercise.

Once you feel you have become independent of nicotine and cigarettes, or you reach your target date, try to take a weekend away from your normal environment. Leave your partially consumed pack or your partial carton at home and try to enjoy yourself. If you live in the city, go to the country; if your home is in the mountains, visit the city. It is only normal to have a twinge of longing for that cigarette, but try not to dwell on that need. Keep busy; try some different foods, or a new activity. It may also be beneficial to avoid places where smoking is prevalent for a few weeks, until you have had a chance to establish your new lifestyle.

Once you have truly kicked your dependence, celebrate it each year. Make the anniversary of the day you finally quit for good "Mike's Day" or "Sally's Day." This is your day. Take it off from work. Do exactly what you want to do. Spend your time with those you want to see; eat the foods you enjoy. Celebrate. You've earned it.

APPENDIX 7

▪

MAKING YOUR OWN
SELF-RELAXATION TAPE

The following relaxation script can be dictated into a tape recorder, either by yourself or by a friend with a soothing voice. You might want to play music in the background. Listen to the tape as frequently as you can. It is a "training" tape, so the more you practice the method, the easier it will get.

Feel free to introduce your own variations into the script. Below is a sample script, which includes a soothing place to be that can be altered to suit your own idea of where that calm, relaxing place might be. Do not listen to the tape or practice these techniques while performing tasks that require mental alertness, such as driving. These techniques are best performed while sitting upright (or slightly reclined) in a comfortable chair with your arms on the armrests and your feet resting on the floor.

If you have had a particularly tense day, or feel more upset than usual, do the following exercise before listening to the tape. Inhale and hold your breath for five seconds. At the same time tighten the muscles of your fists, arms, and chest. Then exhale while releasing your muscles and silently saying, "Let go." Repeat the exercise twice. Do the same tense-relax exercise with your stomach muscles.

Self-Relaxation Tape

(Insert your own name), this is your time to relax. Get into a comfortable position and let yourself become fully supported (pause). . . Give yourself full permission to take this time. . . just for you. There is nothing else you need to do at this time. . . nowhere else you need to be.

Now let yourself take three deep, satisfying breaths (pause ten seconds). . . Allow your eyes to gently close. . . Enjoy the coolness of inhalation and the warmth of exhalation. . . Notice where the coolness seems to enter and the warmth seems to leave your body (pause ten seconds). . . As thoughts occur to you, just let them float away. . . like a passing cloud. Thoughts may drift in. . . but let them pass right on through. . . Concentrate on each soothing breath. . . so automatic. . . so effortless.

Now focus your breath into your belly. . . Imagine a balloon in your belly. . . rising and falling with each breath (pause five seconds). With each rise and fall of the balloon, your belly becomes more relaxed.

Perhaps you will notice an area of tingling or warmth somewhere in your body. . . maybe in your eyes, spreading downward like a soothing wave of calm. . . or maybe from your feet, spreading slowly upwards (pause five seconds). Or maybe there is really no sensation that needs to be noticed at all. As your thinking mind wanders. . . let your inner mind wander about. . . It does not matter just how deeply relaxed you care to go. Enjoy all the feelings that you are producing for yourself.

Now imagine that you are sitting in a safe, relaxing place. . . perhaps somewhere you have been before. . . a scenic beach. . . a lush meadow. . . a sparkling mountain lake. . . Allow yourself to see the vivid colors. . . maybe the rich blue sky. . . or the nearby greenery. . . Hear the sounds. . . those that are near. . . and those that are farther away. . . What do you feel under your feet?. . . Is it grass?. . . or sand?. . . Maybe something else?. . . You might even allow yourself to feel the warm sun soaking into your body. . . so nourishing, so calming. . . Let the healing warmth penetrate into all of the tissues and cells of your body... leaving them as limp and relaxed as a rag doll... Enjoy all of the sights, the sounds, the smells, the feelings... Let yourself really be there... as you let any remaining tension just melt away (pause five seconds)... Make a mental note of this soothing, inner feeling, which you can return to whenever you wish.

Now continue to enjoy those feelings of effortless comfort... of serene, inner calm... as long as you like (pause ten seconds)... and now, if you wish, you can become alert and refreshed by slowly counting to five... At the count of five, you can feel fully refreshed, alert yet inwardly relaxed... One... slowly coming back up... Two... becoming more awake... Three... more alert, refreshed, clear-headed... Four... almost all the way up... Five... wide awake, invigorated, and inwardly relaxed.

GLOSSARY

Acetylcholine—an important neurotransmitter in the body that is responsible for transmission of nerve impulses throughout the parasympathetic branch of the autonomic nervous system.

Aerobic exercise—any prolonged, rhythmical exercise that uses major muscle groups. Aerobic exercises require oxygen and increase heart rate and respiratory rate.

Aerophagia—habitual swallowing of air.

Alimentary canal—all of the organs making up the route taken by food as it passes through the body from the mouth to the anus.

Allergy—an abnormal and individual sensitivity to substances that are usually harmless. Traditionally, allergy occurs when the body's preformed antibodies make contact with the offending substance (the allergen), resulting in the allergic reaction.

Amphetamine—usually a white, crystalline powder that stimulates the nervous system.

Amylase—the enzyme responsible for the breakdown of complex carbohydrates into simpler compounds.

Anemia—a deficiency in the quality or quantity of red blood cells.

Antacid—medication used to neutralize stomach acid.

Antispasmodic—medication used to treat intestinal spasms.

Appendectomy—surgical removal of the appendix.

Appendicitis—inflammation or infection of the appendix. The appendix is a four-inch, dead-end pouch attached to the cecum (the first part of the colon).

Arteriosclerosis—thickening and loss of elasticity of the wall of the arteries, frequently referred to as "hardening of the arteries."

Autonomic nervous system—that branch of the nervous system that works without conscious control. The autonomic nervous system has two subdivisions: the sympathetic system and the parasympathetic system.

Barium—A chalky liquid that is either swallowed or inserted into the rectum during X-ray procedures to outline or contrast the lining of the intestinal tract.

Barium enema (lower GI)—an X-ray examination of the colon. During this exam, barium (a chalky liquid) is inserted into the rectum to contrast and outline the colon.

Beta blocker—the class of medications that block the beta receptors in the body. The beta receptors are activated by the neurotransmitter adrenalin.

Bile—a clear yellow or orange fluid produced by the liver that is concentrated and stored in the gallbladder until needed for digestion. The bile salts help to break up large molecules of fat into smaller molecules that may be absorbed by the body.

Bolus—the soft mass of chewed food that enters the esophagus with each swallow.

Bulking agent—an agent that gives bulk to the stool.

Caffeine—a white powder found naturally in coffee and tea that acts as a stimulant to the central nervous system and as a mild diuretic.

Calisthenics—exercises for developing bodily strength and gracefulness.

Casein—a protein found in milk and other dairy products.

Cholecystectomy—surgical removal of the gallbladder.

Cholecystogram—an X ray of the gallbladder taken after the ingestion of tablets that provide contrast of the gallbladder.

Cholecystokinin—a hormone secreted in the small intestine that stimulates contraction of the gallbladder and the colon.

Chyme—a material produced by the action of gastric secretions on ingested food, which is then discharged from the stomach into the first part of the small intestine, called the duodenum.

Clinical history—a patient/physician interview during which detailed information regarding symptoms and past medical problems is obtained.

Colic—pertaining to the colon. "Colic" usually refers to attacks of abdominal pain that are thought to result from spasms of the intestines. Colic occurs most frequently in infants.

Colon—the part of the large intestine extending from the small intestine to the rectum.

Colonoscopy—endoscopic (see *Endoscopy*) or direct visualization of the entire colon utilizing a fiberoptic scope, referred to as a colonoscope.

Colon polyp—a small, fleshy, mushroom-shaped growth occurring in the colon. Certain types of colon polyps are believed to undergo cancerous transformation if not removed.

Complex carbohydrate—a large molecule consisting of simple carbohydrates or simple sugars linked together. Complex carbohydrates are found in grains, fruits, vegetables, and "starchy" foods (such as bread, rice, pasta), among other foods.

Crohn's disease—a form of inflammatory bowel disease also referred to as regional enteritis, which involves inflammation of the intestinal tract (frequently the last portion of the small intestine, known as the ileum).

Defecation—the elimination of wastes and undigested food as feces from the anus.

Diagnosis—the art or method of identifying or recognizing disease.

Digestion—the process whereby food is broken down into smaller units suitable for absorption into the blood and utilization by the body's individual cells.

Diverticulitis—inflammation of diverticula. Symptoms of diverticulitis may include abdominal pain, usually in the left lower abdomen, and fever.

Diverticulosis—the presence of diverticula.

Diverticulum—a small blind pouch that forms in the wall of the colon.

Duodenum—the first portion of the small intestine, which is usually approximately 10 inches long.

Elimination diet—a diet used for diagnosing food allergies or sensitivities, based on omission of foods that might cause symptoms.

Emulsifier—a substance used to break up and mix two liquids that under ordinary circumstances will not mix—such as oil and water. Detergents act as emulsifiers by breaking up grease, which may then mix with water. Bile acids, produced by the liver, are also emulsifiers, since they aid in digestion by breaking up fats in the intestinal tract, making them suitable for absorption into the bloodstream.

Endorphin—a naturally occurring protein produced in the brain that has a pain-relieving "morphinelike" effect. Among other things, endorphines are thought to mediate the so-called "runner's high."

Endoscopy—the visual examination of the interior structures of the body through a lighted fiberoptic instrument referred to as an endoscope.

Eructation (belching)—the oral ejection of air from the stomach.

Esophageal spasm—a cramplike pain, usually in the center of the chest, produced by spasms of the esophagus.

Esophagogastroduodenoscopy (EGD)—direct observation of the esophagus, stomach, and duodenum through a lighted fiberoptic instrument referred to as an endoscope.

Esophagus—that portion of the alimentary canal that extends from the back of the throat to the stomach. In an average adult, it usually measures 10 to 12 inches long.

Exercise stress test—a continuous monitoring of the heart's electrical activity during exercise to ascertain exercise tolerance and the presence of underlying heart abnormalities provoked by exercise.

Fiber—the undigested portion of fruits, vegetables, and grains. The components of fiber are divided into those that are water soluble (pectins, gums, mucilages, and some hemicelluloses) and those that are insoluble in water (lignins, cellulose, and the remainder of the hemicelluloses).

Fibrocystic breast disease—usually painful, cystic swelling in the breast. The discomfort is usually worse before and during menstrual flow.

Fibromyalgia syndrome (FMS)—a syndrome characterized by a generalized deep muscular aching and associated with fatigue. The disorder is more common in women than men and may be associated with a sleep disturbance.

Fight or flight response—the activation of the sympathetic branch of the autonomic nervous system, preparing one to meet a threat or challenge.

Flatus—gas or air in the stomach or rectum.

Functional disorder—a disorder characterized by abnormal bodily function without a known, identifiable structural disease.

Gallbladder—a saclike structure located under the liver that stores bile. Gallstones may form in the gallbladder, blocking the exit of bile and producing intense pain, usually in the upper abdomen.

Gastroenterologist—a physician with special training in the diganosis and treatment of diseases affecting the digestive system.

Giardiasis—a parasitic infection of the intestinal tract, caused by the *Giardia* protozoa, which produces a diarrheal illness.

Gland—an organ that secretes a specific substance.

Glucose—a simple sugar, also called dextrose; the principal simple sugar in the human body and body fluids.

Gluten—a protein found in wheat and other grains.

H₂ blocker—a class of medications that block the histamine₂ receptors in the body. Most frequently, these medications are used to treat disorders that result from or are made worse by excessive acid secretions in the stomach (for example, peptic ulcer disease).

Hemorrhoid—a mass of dilated veins around the rectum or anus.

Hepatic flexure syndrome—a pain syndrome produced when gas or air accumulates in the upper aspects of the colon on the right side, under the liver.

Hiatal hernia—protrusion of a portion of the stomach through the diaphragm into the chest.

Hydrogen breath test—a test used to determine lactose intolerance as well as other conditions. During the test, samples of expired air are analyzed for hydrogen content.

Hypoglycemia—an abnormally low level of sugar (glucose) in the blood. Symptoms include: headache, rapid heart rate, sweating, nausea, mental confusion, and faint feeling.

Indigestion—failure of digestive function. Indigestion usually refers to acid indigestion (heartburn), which produces burning pains in the chest and may result from eating certain foods, eating too much, or eating too fast.

Inflammation—a tissue response to injury or destruction marked by redness, heat, and/or pain, among other symptoms. The injury may be produced by a variety of means, such as infection, excessive acid, excessive sunlight, or extremes of temperature.

Inflammatory bowel disease (IBD)—those disorders that involve inflammation of the intestinal tract and are often characterized by severe, sometimes bloody diarrhea, abdominal pain, and weight loss.

Insulin—the hormone produced by the pancreas gland that regulates the rate at which the body utilizes carbohydrates. An absolute or relative deficiency of insulin results in the disorder referred to as diabetes.

Internist—a physician specializing in the treatment of adult medical problems. Traditionally, internists have special training in the treatment of diseases that affect the internal organs. An internist is to an adult as a pediatrician is to a child.

Intestinal adhesion—an abnormal fibrous band that develops between internal organs, often after abdominal surgery.

Lactase—the enzyme that is deficient in the intestinal lining of patients with a lactose intolerance.

Lactase enzyme supplement—enzyme supplements that are obtained in liquid or tablet form to treat patients with lactose intolerance.

Lactose intolerance—an inability of the body to metabolize the complex carbohydrate lactose as the result of deficient amounts of lactase enzyme. Symptoms include crampy abdominal pain, diarrhea, bloating, belching, and excessive gas.

Laparotomy—surgery of the abdominal cavity.

Lipase—the enzyme that catalyzes the decomposition of fats into smaller subunits.

Lower esophageal sphincter—the one-way valve between the esophagus and the stomach that ordinarily prevents food from going back up or regurgitating into the esophagus.

Lower GI—See *Barium enema*.

Mastication—the chewing of food; the only voluntary aspect of digestion.

Metabolism—the sum total of the processes and reactions whereby the body utilizes the nutrients absorbed into the bloodstream after food has been digested.

Motility—ability to move spontaneously.

Mucin—a mixture of proteins that is the chief constituent of mucus.

Mucus—the free slime of the mucous membrane, composed of its secretion, mucin, and various salts and body cells.

Nicotine—the substance found in tobacco products that may lead to indigestion, increased blood pressure, and constriction of blood vessels. It has also been linked to heart disease, lung cancer, and other diseases.

Nonulcer dyspepsia—burning "ulcerlike" abdominal pains in the absence of a demonstrable ulcer by X rays or endoscopy.

Palpitation—a heartbeat that is unusually rapid, strong, or irregular.

Pancreas—a large gland located below and behind the stomach. It secretes insulin to help regulate the blood glucose and also secretes various enzymes that aid in the digestive process.

Parasympathetic nervous system—that branch of the autonomic nervous system that normally concerns itself with "energy-conserving" properties. Activation of the parasympathetic nervous system results in, among other things, decreased heart rate, decreased respiratory rate, and increased blood flow to the digestive organs. The major neurotransmitter of the parasympathetic nervous system is acetylcholine.

Peptic ulcer—a sore on the inner part of the stomach or duodenum, thought to result from excessive stomach acid or a breakdown of the mucusal lining of the stomach or duodenum.

Periodontal disease—disease affecting the teeth, gums, and supporting structures.

Peristalsis—the wavelike progression or alternate contraction and relaxation of muscle fibers found in the alimentary tract that serves to propel the contents along.

Placebo—an inactive substance resembling a medication that may be given during experiments to determine psychological effects.

Premenstrual syndrome (PMS)—a syndrome characterized by mood changes, irritability, breast swelling and tenderness, abdominal cramps, and fluid retention that occurs 10 to 14 days before the onset of menstrual flow.

Primary-care physician—usually a family physician, internist, or pediatrician who provides preventive care and treats medical problems when they occur. The primary-care physician makes appropriate referrals to specialists when required.

Proctalgia fugax—intense rectal pain occurring as the result of spasms of the muscles around the anus.

Protease—the enzyme responsible for breaking down proteins into their smaller constituent amino acids.

Purgative—a medicine that produces a purging effect and results in free evacuation of feces.

Radioallergosorbent test (RAST)—a blood test used to determine the presence of antibodies to various substances that may cause allergic reactions.

Radiologist—a medical doctor with specialized training and expertise in X-ray procedures.

Rate of Perceived Exertion (RPE) Scale—a scale that is used when prescribing intensity of exercise and that correlates descriptive terms with numbers.

Rectum—the lowest portion of the large intestine, which stores feces until elimination.

Reflux esophagitis—the regurgitation of acid stomach contents into the esophagus, which produces burning pains frequently referred to as heartburn or indigestion.

Rheumatologist—a physician with special training in treating rheumatologic disease—those diseases that produce pain in the joints or muscles.

Satiety—the state occurring when one feels full or satisfied.

Side effect—a consequence other than that for which a medication is used, especially an adverse effect on another organ system.

Sigmoid exam (sigmoidoscopy)—direct examination of the interior of the sigmoid colon by the use of an endoscope.

Sitz bath—a warm water bath often used to treat conditions of the rectum or vagina. Enough warm water is placed in a tub to just cover the rectal or vaginal area.

Smooth muscle—sheets of muscle fibers found lining hollow structures in the body such as blood vessels, the intestines, bronchial breathing tubes, and the uterus.

Spastic colon—the most frequently used synonym in the past for irritable bowel syndrome (IBS).

Spigelian hernia—a protrusion of the intestinal contents through a weak area in the lower, lateral abdominal wall, usually occurring in women after one or multiple pregnancies.

Splenic flexure syndrome—a pain syndrome produced when gas or air accumulates in the upper aspects of the colon on the left side under the spleen.

Stool specimen—fecal discharge from the bowel that is collected and submitted for laboratory evaluation.

Stress—the experience of strain or tension.

Sympathetic nervous system—that branch of the autonomic nervous system that is also commonly referred to as the "fight or flight" response. This branch of the autonomic nervous system prepares the body to meet a threat or challenge by, among other things, increasing heart rate, increasing respiratory rate, and increasing blood flow to muscles. The major neurotransmitter of the sympathetic nervous system is adrenalin.

Symptom—a recognizable change in a person's physical or mental state, which frequently brings the person to a physician's office.

Syndrome—a group of symptoms or signs that, occurring together, produce a pattern typical of a particular disorder.

Target pulse—the pulse rate that should be ideally maintained for a defined period of time to optimize an aerobic workout. It is usually obtained by subtracting your age from 220 and multiplying by 0.70. (Please refer to Chapter 8, "The Importance of Proper Exercise," for a more detailed discussion.)

Ulcerative colitis—a form of inflammatory bowel disease that involves inflammation of the colon and produces ulcerations or sores. Symptoms consist of severe, sometimes bloody diarrhea, abdominal pain, and weight loss.

Ultrasound—the use of sound waves to produce images of structures within the abdomen.

Upper GI—an X-ray examination of the esophagus, stomach, and duodenum. During this exam, barium (a chalky liquid) is ingested to contrast and outline the esophagus, stomach, and duodenum.

Urinalysis—analysis of urine as an aid in diagnosis.

Villi—the multitudinous fingerlike projections covering the surface of the inner lining of the intestines that are designed to increase the absorptive capabilities of the intestinal tract.

FURTHER READINGS

Jane Brody's Good Food Book by Jane Brody (New York: W.W. Norton & Company, 1985) is a well-researched, comprehensive nutritional guide that also contains healthful recipes.

Cooking Light (Birmingham, AL: Oxmoor House, 1991) is published yearly and contains a variety of easy-to-prepare, nutritious recipes that are "guided by the premise that good health and good food are synonymous." The initial pages contain valuable, up-to-date information about food and fitness.

Time Power by Charles R. Hobbs, Ed.D. (New York: Harper & Row, 1987) is a useful guide for effective time management. The cassette series *Your Time and Your Life*, also by Dr. Hobbs, is available through Day-Timers, Inc., One Day-Timer Plaza, Allentown, PA 18195 ($59.95).

The Relaxation and Stress Reduction Workbook by M.C. Kay (Emeryville, CA: Publisher's Group West, 1988) is an excellent source of information for those who wish to learn the principles of stress management.

A Little Relaxation by Dr. Saul Miller (Pt. Roberts, WA: Hartley & Marks, 1991) offers simple step-by-step instructions for practicing relaxation techniques.

How to Stop Worrying and Start Living by Dale Carnegie (New York: Simon & Schuster, 1984) is a classic that provides insight into how to deal with life's daily trials and tribulations.

The Aerobics Program for Total Well Being by Kenneth H. Cooper, M.D., MPH (New York: Bantam Books, 1982) is an informative guide for developing an individual fitness program.

The Pill Book (New York: Bantam Books, 1990) contains complete information on the most commonly prescribed medications, including drug interactions and side effects.

Natural Health, Natural Medicine by Andrew Weil, M.D. (Boston: Houghton Mifflin Company, 1990) is an excellent book that provides strategies for wellness and self-care. In his book Dr. Weil explores such things as proven home remedies and the healing properties of herbs.

INDEX

Abdominal pain, 2, 18, 25. See also Gas, preventing
  medications for, 163, 165
  preventing, 95
Acetylcholine. See also Autonomic nervous system, 59
  definition of, 192
Adhesions, intestinal, 127–128, 198
Aerophagia, definition of, 23, 192
  results of, 22, 27, 96, 170
Alcohol, digestive effects, 24, 26, 84–85
  in esophagitis, 124
  in exclusion diet, 45, 48
Alimentary canal, 143, 12
  definition of, 192
Allergic reaction, process in, 30–31
  in tests, 142
Allergy, definition of, 192
Anti-anxiety medications, 175–177
Anti-depressants, 102–103, 177–178
  in Fibromyalgia syndrome, 119
Anti-spasmodics, 102, 165
Anti-ulcer medications, 126
  about, 171–173
Appendicitis, 132–133
  definition of, 193
Autonomic nervous system, and stress, 56–60
  in digestion, 13, 22

Barium. See also Upper and Lower gastrointestinal x-ray
  definition of, 193
  enema, 135, 141–142, 193, 198
Belching, 2, 26
Bile, digestive, 15
Bloating, in IBS, 2, 18, 22, 26–27, 32, 53
Bowel infection, 3, 137
Bowel movements, 1, 51
  laxatives for, 93, 168–169
  timing of, 90–93

Caffeine, definition of, 193

digestive effects, 24–26, 33, 45, 124
  using in moderation, 48
Calories, calculating fat, 81
Causes of Irritable Bowel Syndrome symptoms. See Alcohol, Caffeine, Fiber, lack of; Food Sensitivities, Fructose, Lactose, Nicotine, Sorbitol, Stress
Cholecystectomy. See also Gallbladder 136–137, 166
  definition of 15
Cholecystogram, 142
Cholecystokinin, in digestion, 19, 23, 92
Cholelithiasis. See Gallbladder, stones of
Chyme, 127, 128
  role in digestion, 14, 96
Cigarette smoking. See Nicotine
Clinical history, completion of, 151–157
  definition of, 194
  importance of, 6, 148
  questionnaire for, 7–11
Colitis. See Inflammatory bowel disease
Colon cancer, 92, 131–2, 141
  IBS and, 122–123
  testing for, 145
Colonoscopy, 143
  as a diagnostic tool, 130–131, 146
Complex carbohydrates, 14, 97
  in ideal diet, 28–29, 51, 90
Constipation, 2, 18, 25, 102, 104
  medications for, 167–169
  preventing, 92–93
Crohn's disease, 141. See also Inflammatory bowel disease

Dairy products. See Lactose intolerance
Diarrhea, 2, 25, 40
  medications for, 102, 166–167, 175–176
  preventing, 94–95
Diets, and premenstrual syndrome, 115
  diaries of, 36–38, 43, 75–76, 97
  elimination, 30, 39–48

ideal, 28–29, 40
Dietary fiber. See Fiber
Dietician/Nutritionist, 48, 53
    in meal planning, 75–76
Digestion, chewing's role in, 13, 22
Digestive enzymes, 14–15
    supplemental, 174
Diverticula, 145
    129–130
Diverticulosis/Diverticulitis, 141
    129–131
Doctors, choosing, 4–5
    when to seek, 123, 125, 160–161
Duodenal ulcers. See Peptic ulcer disease
Drug side effects, 164. See also individual
    type of medication.

Endoscopy, 158–158. See also
    Sigmoidoscopy 143–144
Endorphins, 67
Eructation. See Belching
Erythrocyte Sedimentation Rate (ESR),
    definition of, 147
Esophageal spasm, 104, 125
Esophagogastroduodenoscopy (EGD),
    144–145
Exercise, 70–73
    before beginning, 68
    benefits of, 67
    importance of, 66
    types of, 69
    stress test, 68

Fiber, 17
    50–55, 184–185
    in diverticulosis, 129–131
    increasing dietary, 90–91, 135, 132
    types of, 101
Fibromyalgia, 3, 103, 114, 117–119
Flatus. See Gas
Food sensitivities, general 17, 30–33, 36,
    42–48
Fructose, definition of 33
    foods containing, 44–45, 79
    sensitivity to, 33–34
    testing for malabsorption of, 147

Gallbladder, 15, 142, 143, 148
    stones of, 136–137
Gas, 2, 26, 32, 40, 53
    preventing, 95–98
    medications for reducing, 169–171
Gastric ulcers. See Peptic ulcer disease
Gastroenterologist, 119
    42, 119–120, 144, 146
    definition of, 4
Giardiasis, 137

Glucose, 51–52
Gluten, 78
    definition of, 41
    foods involved, 44–46

H2 blocker, 104
    definition of 197
Helicobacterpyloris. See Peptic ulcer
    disease
Hemorrhoids, 145
    about, 133–135
    with IBS, 122
Hiatal hernia, with IBS, 122
    with reflux esophagitis, 125
Hydrogen breath test. See Lactose
    intolerance, testing for

Inflammatory bowel disease, 131, 141
    testing for, 147
    versus IBS, 160
International Association for Medical
    Assistance to Travelers, 86
Internist, 5
    about 119–120
Intestinal adhesions. See Adhesions
Intestinal villi, role in digestion, 15
Irritable bowel syndrome. See
    individually listed symptoms
    other names for, ix, 1
    statistical occurrence, 2, 108
    steps to establishing diagnosis of, 3–5,
        158–159
    treatment in general, xii, 23, 101, 159,
        163

Labeling terms, food products, 79–81, 85
Lactase enzyme supplements, in lactose
    intolerance, 32, 146–147, 162, 181
Lactose intolerance, 31–33, 40, 79, 97
    foods involved, 44–46, 182–183
    testing for, 32–48, 146–147, 161
Lactulose, in treating constipation,
    168–169
Laparotomy, for adhesions, 127
Laxatives, 98, 168–169
    in testing, 141
Lower esophageal sphincter (LES),
    definition of, 26
    about, 33, 124
Lower gastrointestinal x-ray. See Barium,
    enema

Mastication. See Digestion, chewing
Maximum predicted heart rate. See also
    Exercise, duration, frequency and
    intensity of
    calculating, 71

Meal planning. See also Labeling terms
  steps in, 74–83
  when eating out, 83–85
  when traveling, 86–87
Medications. See also the type of
    medication: Anti-anxiety, Anti-
    depressant,
  Anti-spasmodic, Anti-ulcer, Digestive
    enzyme, Gas reducers, Laxatives,
  Non-narcotic opioids, Prokinetics
  pregnancy and, 101, 164, 176
Milk products. See Lactose intolerance
Monosodium glutamate, 34, 85

Nicotine, dependence on, 186–188
  digestive effects, 24, 27, 34, 124
Non-narcotic opioids, 102–103
Non-ulcer dyspepsia, 127

Pain. See Abdominal pain
Parasympathetic nervous system. See
    Autonomic nervous system
Peptic ulcer disease, 125–127
  medications for, 165
Peristalsis, 14, 102
  in digestion, 15–16, 18, 128
Polyps, 123, 141, 144. See also colon
    cancer
Premenstrual syndrome, 3, 26
  with IBS, 114–117
Proctalgia fugax, 135–136
Prokinetic agents, 173–174
Psyllium, use as a bulking agent, 54, 101,
    135, 168
Purgative. See laxative

Questionnaire. See Clinical history.

Radioallergosorbent test (RAST),
    definition of, 41
Radiologist, 140
Rate of perceived exertion scale (RPE),
    71–73
Rechallenging, definition of, 39
  in dieting, 41, 47–48

Reflux esophagitis, 123–125
Relaxation techniques. See also Stress,
    managing
  making a tape for, 189–191
  types of, 63–65

Segmental contractions. See Peristalsis
Sigmoidoscopy, in testing, 130–131, 143,
    145–146
Significant others, expected changes,
    111–113
  information for, regarding IBS'ers,
    106–111
Simethicone, 170–171
Sitz baths, 136, 136
Social readjustment rating scan, 56
Sorbitol, definition of 33
  testing for malabsorption of, 147
Spastic colon. See IBS, other names for
Spigelian hernia, 129
Stool sample exam, for diagnosing, 3, 137
  infections identified by, 148, 158
Stress. See also Relaxation techniques
  causing IBS symptoms, 17, 19, 30, 40,
    94–95, 158
  managing of, 61–62, 67, 77, 82–83
  sources and types of, 56–60
Sulfites, 34, 78
Sympathetic nervous system. See
    Autonomic nervous system

Target pulse, determining, 71
Tests. See under individual test name
Tranquilizers, in treating IBS, 103

Ulcerative colitis. See Inflammatory
    bowel disease
Ultrasound, 142–143
Upper gastrointestinal x-ray, as diagnostic
    test, 3, 128, 140–141

Villi. See Intestinal villi.

Yeast, in IBS, 120–121

Dear Reader:

As this book goes to press, my thoughts turn to ways of improving future editions. I have found that reader input is invaluable, and I invite your comments and suggestions. If you would be willing to share some of your personal experiences or helpful tips for other IBS sufferers, please send them to us at the address listed below. Be assured that anonymity will be maintained if your anecdotes are used in future editions.

As IBS is usually a chronic and recurring concern, about which new information is constantly emerging, a quarterly newsletter might be very worthwhile for IBS sufferers. If you would be interested, please send a note indicating so, and your name and address will be kept on file should the interest level be high enough to make this sort of publication a reality.

For health care providers interested in IBS, there is a presentation with slides and notes for IBS sufferers available for purchase.

Please address your inquiries, comments, or suggestions to:

Dr. Gerard Guillory
c/o: MTA
P.O. Box 460832
Aurora, CO 80046

If you are unable to obtain copies of this book from your local bookstore, you may order copies from:

In the U.S.:   Hartley & Marks
                      P.O. Box 147
                      Point Roberts, WA 98281

$11.95 plus $1.50 postage and handling charge.

In Canada: Hartley & Marks
                      3661 West Broadway
                      Vancouver, B.C.
                      V6R 2B8

$14.95 plus $1.50 postage and handling charge.